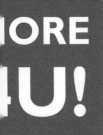 

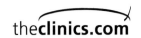

# OBSTETRICS AND GYNECOLOGY CLINICS

# OF NORTH AMERICA

## Cancer Complicating Pregnancy

GUEST EDITOR
Kimberly K. Leslie, MD

CONSULTING EDITOR
William F. Rayburn, MD

December 2005 • Volume 32 • Number 4

**SAUNDERS**

An Imprint of Elsevier, Inc.
PHILADELPHIA   LONDON   TORONTO   MONTREAL   SYDNEY   TOKYO

**W.B. SAUNDERS COMPANY**
*A Division of Elsevier Inc.*

Elsevier, Inc. • 1600 John F. Kennedy Blvd. • Suite 1800 • Philadelphia, PA 19103-2899

http://www.theclinics.com

OBSTETRICS AND GYNECOLOGY
CLINICS OF NORTH AMERICA
December 2005
Editor: Carin Davis

Volume 32, Number 4
ISSN 0889-8545
ISBN 1-4160-2742-4

The ideas and opinions expressed in *Obstetrics and Gynecology Clinics of North America* do not necessarily reflect those of the Publisher. The Publisher does not assume any responsibility for any injury and/or damage to persons or property arising out of or related to any use of the material contained in this periodical. The reader is advised to check the appropriate medical literature and the product information currently provided by the manufacturer of each drug to be administered to verify the dosage, the method and duration of administration, or contraindications. It is the responsibility of the treating physician or other health care professional, relying on independent experience and knowledge of the patient, to determine drug dosages and the best treatment for the patient. Mention of any product in this issue should not be construed as endorsement by the contributors, editors, or the Publisher of the product or manufacturers' claims.

*Obstetrics and Gynecology Clinics of North America* (ISSN 0889-8545) is published quarterly by Elsevier Inc. Corporate and editorial offices: Elsevier, Inc., 1600 John F. Kennedy Blvd., Suite 1800, Philadelphia, PA 19103-2899. Accounting and circulation offices: 6277 Sea Harbor Drive, Orlando, FL 32887-4800. Periodicals postage paid at Orlando, FL 32862, and additional mailing offices. Subscription prices are $180.00 per year for US individuals, $300.00 per year for US institutions, $90.00 per year for US students and residents, $215.00 per year for Canadian individuals, $370.00 per year for Canadian institutions, $245.00 per year for international individuals, $370.00 per year for international institutions and $125.00 per year for Canadian and foreign students/residents. To receive student/resident rate, orders must be accompanied by name of affiliated institution, date of term, and the signature of program/residency coordinator on institution letterhead. Orders will be billed at individual rate until proof of status is received. Foreign air speed delivery is included in all Clinics subscription prices. All prices are subject to change without notice. POSTMASTER: Send address changes to *Obstetrics and Gynecology Clinics of North America*, W.B. Saunders Company, Periodicals Fulfillment, Orlando, FL 32887-4800. **Customer Service: 1-800-654-2452 (US). From outside of the US, call 1-407-345-4000.**

*Obstetrics and Gynecology Clinics of North America* is also published in Spanish by Mc Graw-Hill Interamericana Editores S.A., P.O. Box 5-237, 06500, Mexico; in Portuguese by Reichmann and Affonso Editores, Rio de Janeiro, Brazil; and in Greek by Paschalidis Medical Publications, Athens, Greece.

*Obstetrics and Gynecology Clinics of North America* is covered in *Index Medicus, Excerpta Medica, Current Concepts/Clinical Medicine, Science Citation Index, BIOSIS, CINAHL, and ISI/BIOMED.*

Printed in the United States of America.

## GOAL STATEMENT

The goal of *Obstetrics and Gynecology Clinics of North America* is to keep practicing physicians up to date with current clinical practice in OB/GYN by providing timely articles reviewing the state of the art in patient care.

## ACCREDITATION

The *Obstetrics and Gynecology Clinics of North America* is planned and implemented in accordance with the Essential Areas and Policies of the Accreditation Council for Continuing Medical Education (ACCME) through the joint sponsorship of the University of Virginia School of Medicine and Elsevier. The University of Virginia School of Medicine is accredited by the ACCME to provide continuing medical education for physicians.

The University of Virginia School of Medicine designates this educational activity for a maximum of 60 category 1 credits per year, 15 category 1 credits per issue, toward the AMA Physician's Recognition Award. Each physician should claim only those credits that he/she actually spent in the activity.

The American Medical Association has determined that physicians not licensed in the US who participate in this CME activity are eligible for AMA PRA category 1 credit.

Category 1 credit can be earned by reading the text material, taking the CME examination online at http://www.theclinics.com/home/cme, and completing the evaluation. After taking the test, you will be required to review any and all incorrect answers. Following completion of the test and evaluation, your credit will be awarded and you may print your certificate.

## FACULTY DISCLOSURE/CONFLICT OF INTEREST

The University of Virginia School of Medicine, as an ACCME accredited provider, endorses and strives to comply with the Accreditation Council for Continuing Medical Education (ACCME) Standards of Commercial Support, Commonwealth of Virginia statutes, University of Virginia policies and procedures, and associated federal and private regulations and guidelines on the need for disclosure and monitoring of proprietary and financial interests that may affect the scientific integrity and balance of content delivered in continuing medical education activities under our auspices.

The University of Virginia School of Medicine requires that all CME activities accredited through this institution be developed independently and be scientifically rigorous, balanced and objective in the presentation/discussion of its content, theories and practices.

All authors/editors participating in an accredited CME activity are expected to disclose to the readers relevant financial relationships with commercial entities occurring within the past 12 months (such as grants or research support, employee, consultant, stock holder, member of speakers bureau, etc.). The University of Virginia School of Medicine will employ appropriate mechanisms to resolve potential conflicts of interest to maintain the standards of fair and balanced education to the reader. Questions about specific strategies can be directed to the Office of Continuing Medical Education, University of Virginia School of Medicine, Charlottesville, Virginia.

*The authors/editors listed below have identified no professional or financial affiliations for themselves or their spouse/partner:*

Jehad Barakat, MD; Marianne Berwick, MPH, PhD; Julia Newton Bishop, MD; John D. Deutsch, MD; Jeffrey Dunkelberg, MD, PhD; Timothy J. Hurley, MD; Mehraboon Irani, MD; Christine E. Koil, MS; Kimberly K. Leslie, MD; James McKinnell, MD; Carolyn Y. Muller, MD; William F. Rayburn, MD; Hamid Sayar, MD; Claire F. Verschraegen, MD; and Charles L. Wiggins, PhD.

*The author listed below identified the following professional or financial affiliations for himself, his spouse/partner:*
**Harriet O. Smith, MD** owns stock in Johnson & Johnson, Pfizer, Wyeth, and Wachovia.

*The authors listed below have not provided disclosure for themselves or their spouse/partner:*
Laurence A. Cole, PhD; Ernest Kohorn, MD; Carol A. Lange, PhD; and Catherine Lhomme, MD.

*Disclosure of discussion of non-FDA approved uses for pharmaceutical products and/or medical devices:* **The University of Virginia School of Medicine, as an ACCME provider, requires that all faculty presenters identify and disclose any "off label" uses for pharmaceutical and medical device products. The University of Virginia School of Medicine recommends that each physician fully review all the available data on new products or procedures prior to instituting them with patients.**

## TO ENROLL

To enroll in the *Obstetrics and Gynecology Clinics of North America* Continuing Medical Education program, call customer service at 1-800-654-2452 or visit us online at www.theclinics.com/home/cme. The CME program is available to subscribers for an additional fee of $195.00

# CONSULTING EDITOR

**WILLIAM F. RAYBURN, MD,** Seligman Professor and Chair, Department of Obstetrics and Gynecology, University of New Mexico Health Sciences Center, Albuquerque, New Mexico

# GUEST EDITOR

**KIMBERLY K. LESLIE, MD,** Professor and Chief of Obstetrics, Division of Maternal-Fetal Medicine, Department of Obstetrics and Gynecology; Co-Director, Women's Cancer Program, Cancer Research and Treatment Center, University of New Mexico Health Sciences Center, Albuquerque, New Mexico

# CONTRIBUTORS

**JEHAD BARAKAT, MD,** Division of Gastroenterology and Hepatology, Department of Internal Medicine, University of New Mexico Health Sciences Center, Albuquerque, New Mexico

**MARIANNE BERWICK, PhD, MPH,** Professor and Chief, Division of Epidemiology, Department of Internal Medicine, University of New Mexico School of Medicine; Head, Epidemiology and Cancer Prevention, University of New Mexico Cancer Research and Treatment Center, Albuquerque, New Mexico

**JULIA A. NEWTON BISHOP, MD,** Professor of Dermatology, Genetic Epidemiology Division, Cancer Research, St. James University Hospital, Leeds, United Kingdom

**LAURENCE A. COLE, PhD,** Professor, Division of Women's Health Research, Department of Obstetrics and Gynecology, University of New Mexico Health Sciences Center, Albuquerque, New Mexico

**JOHN DEUTSCH, MD,** Division of Gastroenterology, St. Mary's Duluth Clinic, Duluth, Minnesota

**JEFFREY C. DUNKELBERG, MD, PhD,** Division of Gastroenterology and Hepatology, Department of Internal Medicine, University of New Mexico Health Sciences Center, Albuquerque, New Mexico

**TIMOTHY J. HURLEY, MD,** Assistant Professor, Division of Maternal and Fetal Medicine, Department of Obstetrics and Gynecology, University of New Mexico Health Science Center; Co-director, The Mother Baby Unit, University of Mew Mexico Health Science Center, Albuquerque, New Mexico

**MEHRABOON S. IRANI, MD,** Medical Director, Tricore Laboratory, Division of Haematology, Department of Pathology, Presbyterian Hospital, Albuquerque, New Mexico

**ERNEST KOHORN, MD,** Professor Emeritus, Department of Obstetrics and Gynecology, Yale University School of Medicine, New Haven, Connecticut

**CHRISTINE KOIL, MS,** Instructor and Genetic Counselor, Division of Maternal-Fetal Medicine, University of New Mexico Health Sciences Center, Albuquerque, New Mexico

**CAROL A. LANGE, PhD,** Associate Professor of Medicine, Departments of Medicine and Pharmacology, University of Minnesota, Minneapolis, Minnesota

**KIMBERLY K. LESLIE, MD,** Professor and Chief of Obstetrics, Division of Maternal-Fetal Medicine, Department of Obstetrics and Gynecology; Co-Director, Women's Cancer Program, Cancer Research and Treatment Center, University of New Mexico Health Sciences Center, Albuquerque, New Mexico

**CATHERINE LHOMME, MD,** Professor of Medicine, Institut Gustave Roussy, Villejuif, France

**JAMES V. MCKINNELL, MD,** Assistant Professor, Division of Oncology, and Haematology, Department of Pediatrics, University of New Mexico Health Science Center, Albuquerque, New Mexico

**CAROLYN Y. MULLER, MD,** Associate Professor and Chief, Division of Gynecologic Oncology, Department of Obstetrics and Gynecology, University of New Mexico Health Sciences Center, Albuquerque, New Mexico

**WILLIAM F. RAYBURN, MD,** Seligman Professor and Chair, Department of Obstetrics and Gynecology, University of New Mexico Health Sciences Center, Albuquerque, New Mexico

**HAMID SAYAR, MD,** Fellow in Medical Oncology and Hematology; Cancer Research and Treatment Center, Division of Hematology Oncology, University of New Mexico, Albuquerque, New Mexico

**HARRIET O. SMITH, MD,** Professor, Division of Gynecologic Oncology, Department of Obstetrics and Gynecology, University of New Mexico Health Sciences Center, Albuquerque, New Mexico

**CLAIRE F. VERSCHRAEGEN, MD,** Associate Professor of Medicine, Cancer Research and Treatment Center, Division of Hematology Oncology, University of New Mexico, Albuquerque, New Mexico

**CHARLES L. WIGGINS, PhD,** Assistant Professor, Division of Epidemiology, Department of Internal Medicine, University of New Mexico School of Medicine; Director and Principal Investigator, New Mexico Tumor Registry, Albuquerque, New Mexico

# CONTENTS

and the effect of pregnancy on lifetime risk for breast cancer in the general population and for women with mutations in *BRCA1* and *BRCA2* are also discussed.

## Malignant Melanoma in Pregnancy
Charles L. Wiggins, Marianne Berwick, and Julia A. Newton Bishop

This article provides a concise overview of issues relating to melanoma and pregnancy, including pregnancy-associated risk and prognosis, and briefly summarizes results from relevant reports that have been published in recent years. The bulk of evidence amassed over the past half century suggests that pregnancy does not significantly affect the risk of developing malignant melanoma. Further, pregnancy does not seem adversely to influence overall survival from the disease. Most studies found no difference in overall survival between pregnant and nonpregnant women with melanoma. Recent reports from large-scale, population-based studies support these conclusions.

## Malignant Adnexal Masses in Pregnancy
Hamid Sayar, Catherine Lhomme, and Claire F. Verschraegen

Ovarian tumors during pregnancy are very rare; however, a cancer diagnosis causes distress to the couple. Reassurance is paramount, and the first consideration should be given to the safety of the mother. If both mother and fetus can be preserved, treatment to minimize the risks to both should be planned accordingly. It is imperative to care for the patient with a multidisciplinary team that includes a high-risk obstetrician, a gynecologic oncologist, and a medical oncologist specialized in gynecologic cancers.

## Hematologic Malignancies in Pregnancy
Timothy J. Hurley, James V. McKinnell, and Mehraboon S. Irani

Hematologic malignancies complicating pregnancy are uncommon, but a delay in diagnosis or treatment can mean the difference between life and death. It is the responsibility of the obstetrician, nurse-midwife, or nurse practitioner to maintain a high index of suspicion when patients present with unexplained lymphadenopathy or protracted constitutional symptoms. Management of these patients requires a multifaceted team from the oncology, pediatrics, and obstetrics services. With most hematologic cancers now requiring multiagent chemotherapy for optimal survival, the patient, her family, and her physicians are often faced with what seems to be a Faustian dilemma. Most infants exposed in utero to multiagent chemotherapy, however, seem to suffer no long-term detrimental consequences.

# FORTHCOMING ISSUES

# RECENT ISSUES

---

## The Clinics are now available online!
### http://www.theclinics.com

---

ELSEVIER
SAUNDERS

Obstet Gynecol Clin N Am
32 (2005) xiii–xiv

OBSTETRICS AND
GYNECOLOGY
CLINICS
OF NORTH AMERICA

Foreword

# Cancer Complicating Pregnancy

This issue of the *Obstetrics and Gynecology Clinics of North America*, prepared by Guest Editor Dr. Kimberly Leslie, deals with cancer complications in pregnancy. The most common malignancies associated with pregnancy are those of the genital tract, breast, and malignant melanoma. According to the National Center for Health Statistics, cancer is the second leading cause of death in women 25 to 44 years of age. Malignancies during pregnancy are not rare and account for about 5% of all maternal deaths.

This multidisciplinary group of authors provides a comprehensive overview in assisting the obstetrician in caring for persons afflicted with cancer who are either contemplating or have been diagnosed to be pregnant. Although her care may need to be modified, she should not be penalized for being pregnant. The following questions are noteworthy for our consideration:

- If the malignancy exists before conception, how should the patient be counseled about birth control and about future child bearing?
- Is pregnancy advisable after cancer treatment?
- Should the pregnancy be terminated because it represents an obstacle for effective cancer therapy?
- Does pregnancy affect progression of the disease?
- What risk does cancer or its treatment pose to the developing fetus?

Answers to these questions will be addressed in this issue for specific malignancies involving the hemopoetic system, gastrointestinal system, melanomas, breast, genital tract (ovary, cervix), and trophoblast disorders.

In addition, this issue addresses controversies surrounding treatment during pregnancy. Surgery for suspected or proven cancer may be indicated for diagnostic, staging, or therapeutic reasons. Extra-abdominal procedures and most intraperitoneal operations that do not interfere with the reproductive tract are usually well tolerated by the mother and fetus. Unlike diagnostic radiographic procedures, therapeutic radiation may result in significant fetal exposure to ionizing radiation. The necessity of therapeutic radiation raises issues such as abortion, teratogenesis, and fetal sequelae. Despite pregnancy, chemotherapy is often recommended for a variety of hemopoetic and lymphatic malignancies and as adjunctive therapy to surgery or radiation. If fertility is not impaired, questions arise regarding increased risk of abortion, fetal chromosomal damage, fetal anomalies, restricted fetal growth, and risk of malignancy in future offspring.

It is our desire that this issue attract the attention of providers caring for women of reproductive age with a malignancy. Practical information provided herein will hopefully aid in the development and implementation of more specific and individualized treatment programs.

William F. Rayburn, MD
*Department of Obstetrics and Gynecology*
*University of New Mexico*
*MSC 10 5580*
*1 University of New Mexico*
*Albuquerque, NM 87131-0001, USA*
*E-mail address:* wrayburn@salud.unm.edu

OBSTETRICS AND
GYNECOLOGY
CLINICS
OF NORTH AMERICA

Obstet Gynecol Clin N Am
32 (2005) xv–xvi

Preface

# Cancer Complicating Pregnancy

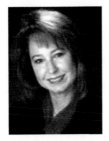

Kimberly K. Leslie, MD
*Guest Editor*

Cancer is the leading cause of death among women aged 35 to 54. As childbearing among older parturients increases, so likely will the incidence of cancer in pregnancy. Currently, cancer complicates one in 1000 pregnancies. The management of pregnant women with cancer presents a major challenge to the care-giving team: the risks and benefits of treatment (and withholding treatment) must be weighed for both the mother and the fetus.

The purpose of this issue of the *Obstetrics and Gynecology Clinics of North America* is to review the known literature on the diagnosis and management of cancer during pregnancy. Cervical cancer is the most frequent malignant neoplasm in pregnancy, followed by breast cancer and melanoma. Other malignancies seen more rarely are ovarian cancer, leukemia, lymphoma, and colorecatal cancer. In addition, choriocarcinoma remains a problem and a potential diagnostic dilemma for clinicians. We have included manuscripts on these specific cancer sites as well as information on how to follow women with persistently low-positive human chorionic gonadotropin levels. To assist in the choice of therapeutic regimens for cancers during pregnancy, an article on the use of chemotherapy is also provided.

One interesting question to consider is whether pregnancy accelerates carcinogenesis or tumor progression, particularly for hormone-related cancers. We deal with that issue in the articles included herein to the extent possible given the heterogeneity of the literature addressing the question. However, for many

0889-8545/05/$ – see front matter © 2005 Elsevier Inc. All rights reserved.
doi:10.1016/j.ogc.2005.11.001

*obgyn.theclinics.com*

tumor sites, it does appear that pregnant women present at a more advanced stage compared with age-matched, nonpregnant patients. Whether a causal relationship between pregnancy per se and advanced stage or poor outcome can be assigned remains a topic of debate. Nevertheless, it is likely that clinicians will encounter a disproportionate number of women who have advanced cancers in pregnancy that will necessitate aggressive management to achieve a cure. We hope that these articles will assist clinicians in treating their patients and will positively impact the standard of care provided to pregnant women who have cancer.

Kimberly K. Leslie, MD
*Department of Obstetrics and Gynecology*
*University of New Mexico Health Science Center*
*2211 Lomas Boulevard NE, MSC10 5580*
*Albuquerque, NM 87131, USA*
*E-mail address:* kleslie@salud.unm.edu

ELSEVIER
SAUNDERS

Obstet Gynecol Clin N Am
32 (2005) 533–546

OBSTETRICS AND
GYNECOLOGY
CLINICS
OF NORTH AMERICA

# Cervical Neoplasia Complicating Pregnancy

## Carolyn Y. Muller, MD*, Harriet O. Smith, MD

*Division of Gynecologic Oncology, Department of Obstetrics and Gynecology,
University of New Mexico Health Sciences Center, 1 University of New Mexico, MSC 10 5580,
Albuquerque, NM 87131, USA*

Cervical cancer is the most common malignancy diagnosed during pregnancy, because it is the only cancer routinely screened for during gestation. The incidence is 0.45 to 1 per 1000 live births in the United States, with carcinoma in situ occurring in 1 in 750 pregnancies [1]. Cervical cancer is often detected in the preinvasive or early invasive stage, because pregnancy allows an opportunity for early detection that may be otherwise missed in nonpregnant women who ignore global screening recommendations. Traditional signs and symptoms of invasive cervical cancer can often be misinterpreted as common symptoms of pregnancy (vaginal spotting or discharge, postcoital bleeding, pain) with subtle early invasive cancer mistaken for a pregnancy-induced cervical ectropion, cervical decidualization, or other exaggerated changes of pregnancy [2,3]. A larger lesion may not be appreciated because of other anatomic changes in pregnancy. If not considered on the differential diagnosis, a false-negative Pap smear may delay diagnosis even further. On rare occasion, an unrecognized invasive cervical cancer is a cause of intrapartum hemorrhage resulting in cesarean delivery and a "cut through" cesarean hysterectomy, an intervention that can have an unfortunate impact on subsequent treatment and prognosis of the new mother [4,5].

Once diagnosed, invasive cervical cancer in pregnancy raises many issues necessitating a well-coordinated multidisciplinary approach to therapy. The timing of cancer diagnosis within the gestation dictates available options for treatment. Often, a delicate balance ensues between the welfare of the mother and fetus. Additionally, conflict on moral and ethical grounds may occur between the patient and family and the health care providers introducing more stress regarding

* Corresponding author.
*E-mail address:* cmuller@salud.unm.edu (C.Y. Muller).

the decision-making process [6]. In general, the treatment principals of cervical disease during pregnancy are not significantly different than that within the nonpregnant state. In addition, pregnancy does not seem to alter the biology of the tumor when compared with the nonpregnant state stage for stage. This article addresses the diagnosis and management of preinvasive and invasive cervical disease during pregnancy. In addition, this article highlights some of the impact of cervical cancer treatment on future fertility and treatment [7].

## Human papillomavirus infection in pregnancy

Human papillomavirus (HPV) is involved in nearly all squamous cell and most adenocarcinoma preinvasive and invasive disease of the cervix [8]. HPV is the most common sexually transmitted infection affecting tens of millions of women in the United States [9]. The peak incidence of infection occurs after sexual debut and globally in the third decade of life, a time of maximal reproductive potential [9]. The prevalence of HPV in the United States decreases with age as does fecundity. HPV infection and HPV-related disease is an expected finding in the pregnant patient. Both oncogenic and nononcogenic HPV infections can complicate pregnancy. Oncogenic HPV infection can lead to abnormal cervical cytology determined during pregnancy and requires diagnostic procedures and treatment if indicated. HPV 16 and 18 are the most common oncogenic HPV subtypes found in women at this age regardless of gravity [9,10]. Nononcogenic HPV infections can cause visible condyloma within the entire lower genital tract. These condyloma can undergo rapid proliferation during pregnancy in response to the changing hormonal milieu leading to local symptoms and, on rare occasion, cause laryngeal papillomatosis and other condylomatous changes in the infant [11,12]. The management and treatment of condyloma is beyond the scope of this article.

This article addresses the issues of HPV infection during pregnancy as it relates to cervical dysplasia and cancer risk. The most common misconception is that the relative immunosuppressive state of pregnancy causes an HPV infection to be more aggressive during pregnancy. To date, there is no credible evidence that suggests a different natural history of HPV infection in the gravid state [7,13]. Age for age, the prevalence of HPV in the lower genital tract is comparable between pregnant and nonpregnant women, with a baseline rate of 20% to 30% [10,14,15]. Similarly, most ASCUS cytology and lowgrade and highgrade squamous intraepithelial lesion (LSIL and HSIL) Pap smears show high rates of oncogenic HPV infection [16]. There is no difference between subtypes of infection or multiple simultaneous infections between pregnant and nonpregnant women [17]. Cervical dysplasia risk, persistence, and progression or clearance of disease are discussed later. To date, there is no evidence that the effects of pregnancy modify the infectivity rate, prevalence, or persistence of HPV infections.

# Managing the abnormal Pap smear in pregnancy

Pregnancy is an ideal opportunity to screen for cervical neoplasia. Unless the first presentation to the health care system is during labor, women have the opportunity to undergo at least one Pap smear screen during gestation. In cases with optimal prenatal and postnatal care, women have undergone two or more Pap smears within a 12-month time frame. Recommendations for Pap smear screening include at first prenatal visit and again at the 6-week postpartum visit. Less endocervical cells and more cases of dysplasia have been reported in postpartum Pap smears compared with antepartum Pap smears, supporting the importance of this strategy [18]. The safety and superiority of the endocervical brush as a collection device has been documented in numerous studies and has been the accepted practice for nearly a decade [19–22]. Further advances in Pap smear screening include the movement toward liquid-based cytology. The latter has been shown to have a lower false-negative rate and is ideal for necessary reflex HPV testing [23,24]. Test performance in the pregnant population is lacking, however, for most new Pap smear technologies. There are no reliable data to suggest any additional difference between conventional or liquid-based Pap smears from that measured in the nonpregnant comparative studies, because studies solely in pregnant patients or amply stratified for pregnancy are lacking. The physiology of pregnancy alters cervicovaginal cellular morphology [1,13]. It is important to communicate the gravid state on the history form accompanying the Pap smear, because subtle changes in pregnancy may lead to false-positive results, especially if the history of the pregnant state is unknown to the cytopathologist.

The incidence of abnormal Pap smears in pregnancy is dependent on the population undergoing screening, but may be as high as 5% to 8% in university-based higher-risk populations [25]. Interpretation of the Pap smear in pregnancy and the nonpregnant state complies with the 2001 Bethesda guidelines [26]. With appropriate collection devices and trained health care providers, unsatisfactory Pap smears are less common as the transformation zone undergoes relative migration onto the ectocervix. But when it occurs, the Pap smear should be repeated. All abnormal Pap smears should be evaluated while complying with the same algorithm used in the nonpregnant state [26]. Differences or special issues related to managing the abnormal Pap smear during pregnancy are summarized as follows [26]:

- Refer to expert colposcopist experienced in colposcopy in pregnancy
- Manage according to 2001 Bethesda Guidelines
- HIV-positive women with any ASCUS should undergo expert colposcopy
- Do not perform ECC in pregnancy
- Do not repeat Pap smear less than 6 weeks postpartum

Reflex HPV testing is appropriate for ASCUS Pap smears and colposcopic examination reserved for ASCUS HPV-positive results. Colposcopy should be considered for HIV gravidas with any ASCUS Pap smear [27]. All LSIL and HSIL Pap tests require colposcopic examination [26]. AGUS Pap smears are more difficult to manage, because endocervical curettage is contraindicated in pregnancy [26]. Colposcopy and directed biopsy should be performed in these cases. Diagnostic cervical conization should be reserved for patients only if there is a significant concern for occult malignancy.

## Performing colposcopy in the pregnant patient

The principles of colposcopy pertain to all women regardless of the gravid state. The challenge of performing an adequate colposcopic examination is related to pregnancy changes of the cervix: increased friability caused by relative eversion of the columnar epithelium, cervical distortion from a low-riding fetal head, early effacement, and obstruction of visualization by the mucus plug [1,3]. Special considerations for colposcopy in the pregnant patient are as follows [26]:

- Expert colposcopist should perform the evaluation
- Unsatisfactory examinations may be satisfactory in 6 to 12 weeks or by 20 weeks
- Limit biopsy to worse visible area
- Prepare for increased biopsy site bleeding
- Re-evaluate lesion with Pap smear or colposcopy every 8 to 12 weeks
- Only perform repeat biopsy if the lesion worsens
- Recommend excisional biopsy only if concerned about invasive cancer

It is important that the health care provider performing the colposcopic examination be skilled in performing the test in pregnant women. An unsatisfactory colposcopy may be encountered in the early gestation, but a repeat colposcopy every 4 weeks or within 6 to 12 weeks may allow time for migration of the transformation zone to the ectocervix, allowing a satisfactory examination [3]. Economos and coworkers [25] have found all colposcopies to be satisfactory by 20 gestational weeks.

The characteristics and accuracy of colposcopic detection of both low- and high-grade intraepithelial lesions are similar in both pregnant and nonpregnant women [7]. Examples of LSIL and HSIL in pregnancy lesions are shown in (Figs. 1 and 2), respectively. Such characteristics as acetowhite changes, punctuations, mosaic pattern, and atypical vessels are similar in the pregnant and nonpregnant state. Careful evaluation within everted glandular crypts may be more time consuming, but glandular lesions are more likely to be apparent. Lesions off the cervical portio or in the upper vaginal apex may be more difficult to visualize because of a wider squamocolumnar junction and increased vaginal laxity. Gentle traction on the cervix with a cotton tip swab can be helpful. A confirmatory biopsy to be taken at the most worrisome areas is recommended, although on occasion an expert colposcopist may be comfortable documenting

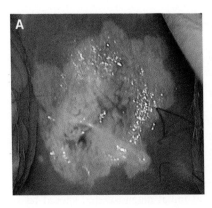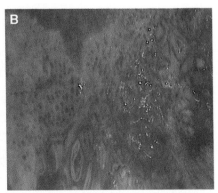

Fig. 1. Colposcopic images of the transformation zone of the cervix at 26 weeks' gestation. The referral Pap smear was atypical squamous cells of undetermined significance (ASCUS) with reflex high-risk HPV identified. Biopsy confirmed CIN1. (*A*) Acetowhite changes involving entire transformation zone (original magnification ×7.5). (*B*) Punctations and early mosaic pattern are seen (3% acetic acid stain, original magnification ×15). (Courtesy of Alan Waxman, MD, Albuquerque, NM.)

the fully visualized lesion with close surveillance without biopsy. Biopsies are more prone to bleed during pregnancy but can be controlled with silver nitrate, Monsel's solution, or local pressure. If needed a careful stitch can be placed at the site of bleeding, but this is rarely needed. Several studies have showed no significant complications from punch biopsies at the time of colposcopy [25,28,29]. Endocervical curettage should not be performed in pregnancy. Repeat colposcopy is required in most cases with intraepithelial lesions, as discussed in the next section.

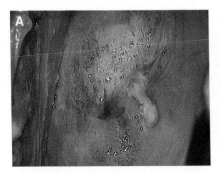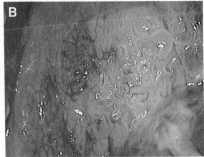

Fig. 2. Colposcopic images of the transformation zone of the cervix at 18 weeks' gestation. The referral Pap smear was highgrade squamous intraepithelial lesion (HSIL). Glandular eversion and increased vascularity of pregnancy make it difficult to see extensive mosaic vascular pattern within the transformation zone. Biopsy confirmed CIN2 with glandular extension. (*A*) 3% acetic acid stain, original magnification ×7.5. (*B*) 3% acetic acid stain, original magnification ×15. (Courtesy of Alan Waxman, MD, Albuquerque, NM.)

## Management of cervical dysplasia in pregnancy

In general, cervical intraepithelial lesions should be managed as if the patient were not pregnant. Unless invasive disease is expected, however, conservative management and follow-up throughout the gestation is strongly recommended, because it is an exceptional case that develops invasive cancer within such a short time frame. In one report, overall the risk of progression from CIN1 to ≥ CIN3 is 1% per year and from CIN2 to ≥ CIN3 is 16% over 2 years [30]. Low-grade lesions have no significant risk of progressing to cancer within the gestational period. Repeat cytology and colposcopy with rebiopsy only if the lesion worsens is the rule. The frequency of repeat evaluation is dependent on the time in the gestation of initial diagnosis and should be at the discretion of the physician managing the evaluations. Guidelines are to repeat the Pap smear and colposcopy every 8 to 12 weeks [1]. Documented high-grade intraepithelial lesions should be monitored carefully throughout the pregnancy with repeat cytology and colposcopy in a similar fashion. Postpartum cytology and colposcopy should be performed no sooner than 6 weeks postpartum. Patient counseling regarding need for follow-up and possible treatment of persistent disease is important, because nearly 30% of patients are expected to be lost to follow-up [18]. Regression of both low- and high-grade lesions occurs after delivery. Controversy still exists as to whether vaginal delivery has a greater impact in allowing lesion regression [31–33]. In most studies, low-grade lesions are more apt to regress (as is true in the nonpregnant state) and are reported as high as 36% to 70% [32,34,35]. The regression rates for high-grade lesions and carcinoma in situ is 48% to 70%, respectively, with an overall incidence of progression to cancer of 0% to 0.4% [33,34]. Persistent or progressive disease diagnosed in the postpartum period should be treated according to the algorithm used in the nonpregnant state.

Cervical conization during gestation is reserved only for suspicion of invasive cancer [26]. Classic conization in pregnancy can be disastrous, resulting in significant hemorrhage (> 500 mL) necessitating vaginal packing, transfusion, hospitalization, miscarriage, fetal loss, and increased perinatal death rates. The risk of significant hemorrhage increases with each trimester of the gestation (< 1%, 5%, 10%, respectively) [3]. Spontaneous fetal loss in the first trimester after conization has been reported as high as 18%, but this compares with average loss rate of 10% to 15% of all first-trimester gestations [28]. Perinatal death rate postconization is reported close to 5%, again in line with overall death rate [28]. Delivery before 37 weeks is caused by subsequent chorioamnionitis occurring weeks after conization, and has been reported in up to 12% of cases [3]. If absolutely indicated, a cone biopsy is best performed between 14 and 20 weeks gestation with or without cervical cerclage. Some advocate cerclage to control bleeding [36]. Conizations should not be performed within 4 weeks of anticipated delivery, because cervical healing is not complete and hemorrhage is likely to ensue at the time of labor and delivery. In lieu of a classic cone biopsy, some advocate "wedge biopsies" or "coin-shaped resections," which provide enough tissue to make the diagnosis while limiting the morbidity associated with a full cone resection [3,7]. If a full conization is warranted, a conization-cerclage technique has been advocated by others [36]. In a desired pregnancy, it is most acceptable to manage expected microinvasive or early invasive carcinoma conservatively, because even 24-week delay in treatment has not been associated with poorer maternal outcomes [37–39]. Each case should be individualized, and unless early termination is desired, any decision to proceed with any kind of conization should be made in a multidisciplinary effort to weigh risks to the mother and the fetus. Conization should be performed only if the results alter the desired treatment. If there is any doubt regarding the appropriateness of this procedure, referral to an expert is warranted.

## Diagnosis and management of invasive cervix cancer

The diagnosis of invasive cervical cancer during pregnancy brings much angst to the patient, family, obstetrician-gynecologist, and other health care providers. Although most cancer cases are diagnosed at an early stage, difficult decisions are needed that impact both the mother and the fetus, which may be in conflict [6]. There is significant evidence that delay in treatment of early stage cancer is not likely to have a deleterious effect on the mother, and that delay of treatment until fetal maturity in a desired pregnancy is a reasonable course of action [39–42]. In more advanced-stage disease, special issues regarding imaging and treatment of the gravid patient can be complicated, and little data are available to guide adequate counseling.

Most women diagnosed with cervical cancer during pregnancy are found to have early stage disease. Microinvasive carcinoma (FIGO stage IA1 and IA2) and visible lesions limited to the cervix (stage IB1 and IB2) complicating pregnancy have been studied extensively under the category of early stage disease [43]. Decisions regarding timing of treatment and delivery are weighted by the trimester in which the diagnosis is made and more importantly the desirability of the pregnancy for the affected woman and her family. Once fetal viability is established, by the third trimester there is little doubt that the risk-benefit ratio favors delaying treatment until fetal lung maturation, because 6- to 12-week delays in all early stage disease has not been shown to worsen overall prognosis or survival in the mother [37–39]. This strategy minimizes fetal morbidity and mortality, NICU days, and all of the chronic complications of prematurity. In these cases, working with a multidisciplinary team including the obstetrician or maternal fetal medicine specialist guides recommendations regarding corticosteroid administration to accelerate fetal lung maturity, timing of amniocentesis to document lung maturity, and mode of delivery. Vaginal delivery is relatively contraindicated when a gross tumor is present (IB), because poorer maternal outcomes have been described and tumor implantation has been found in episiotomy sites [3,44,45]. Cesarean radical hysterectomy with pelvic lymphadenectomy should be scheduled with coordination of the multidisciplinary teams

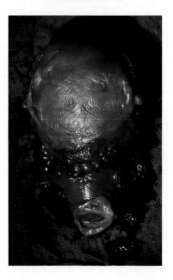

Fig. 3. Surgical specimen after cesarean radical hysterectomy with ovarian preservation. Delivery of a viable fetus was followed by a type III radical hysterectomy. A low transverse incision was made well above the cervix. Vertical hysterotomy incisions are also appropriate to avoid inadvertent incisions into tumor or an effaced cervix.

(Fig. 3). Blood loss and transfusion requirements are greater than in the non-pregnant or early pregnant states [46].

Invasive cervical cancer diagnosed within the first and second trimesters can be a bit more challenging. A recommended algorithm is shown in Fig. 4. Counseling regarding gestations less than 20 weeks (before any definition of fetal viability) is easier than when the diagnosis and impending treatment occurs within the gray zone of fetal viability (22 to 24 weeks). This introduces additional ethical and State issues regarding means of fetal termination, which is beyond the scope of this article. The key two management issues are accurate gestational dating and maternal desire for the pregnancy. If the gestation is ≤ 20 weeks and the pregnancy is undesired, termination can ensue followed by appropriate treatment. If enough data are known to warrant proper surgical intervention, treatment can occur simultaneously as in type II or type III radical hysterectomy with pelvic lymphadenectomy leaving the fetus in situ for stages IA2 or IB cervical cancer. If the extent of the disease is not known, then termination should be completed and further evaluation performed, such as cervical cone biopsy for anticipated microinvasive carcinoma (see Fig. 4).

Within the past decade, changes in the clinical classification of cervical tumors occurred during the FIGO 1994 meeting in Montreal. Stage IB tumors are now stratified into stage IB1 (maximal diameter ≤ 4 cm) and stage IB2 (maximal diameter > 4 cm) [43]. Nearly all prior retrospective series evaluating delay in treatment and maternal outcomes in stage IB patients evaluated cases before this staging distinction. Recent Gynecologic Oncology Group data report an 88% likelihood of requiring either adjuvant radiation or radiation plus

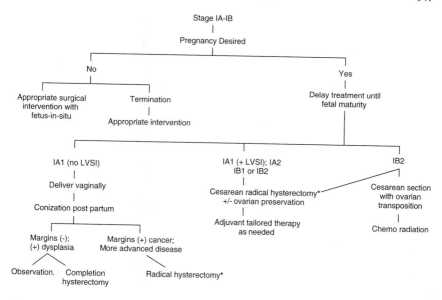

Fig. 4. An algorithm for treatment options in patients with early stage invasive cervical cancer diagnosed less than 20 weeks' gestation.

chemotherapy in patients with IB2 tumors when following adjuvant therapy recommendations for intermediate- and high-risk surgically managed disease [47]. With survival rates in this group comparable with stage IIB cervical cancer patients, primary chemoradiation is an option and can be instituted immediately if the pregnancy is not desired. Radiation therapy induces abortion with an average of 35 to 40 Gy, at a median of 20 to 24 days (or longer if started in the second trimester) [7,48]. There are no data to date that combined chemoradiation alters time to abortion in these patients. Hysterotomy is not recommended unless necessary. Ovarian function ceases after >10 Gy, and may lead to more symptom from both pregnancy and hormonal withdrawal during treatment [49]. Tailored surgery followed by adjuvant radiation with or without chemotherapy allows ovarian transposition and preservation of ovarian function in these women and should be considered. To date, there are no data to suggest superiority in tailored therapy versus primary chemoradiation in IB2 lesions diagnosed in pregnancy. Decisions should take into account individual risks of morbidity and personal preference.

Advanced cervical cancer is rarely encountered in pregnancy, but when discovered can lead to very difficult decisions. The safety of delayed therapy is not clear in this group of patients, although one small series by Sood and coworkers [48] suggests no difference in prognosis with delay for fetal maturity. Some women, however, choose to maintain the gestation at the potential cost to their own health. Evaluation of local and distant disease should proceed cautiously, with MRI the image modality of choice during gestation [50]. There is no curative treatment for stage IVB disease, and palliative measures and fetal issues likely should supersede. There are no case reports of metastatic cervix cancer to the fetus or placenta. Treatment for stage IIB-IVA should be directed toward curative intent, and maternal outcome should weigh greater than fetal well-being. Chemoradiation is the mainstay of therapy and should be initiated promptly. Nonviable fetuses abort with radiation. There are no data to suggest fetal loss occurs sooner with chemoradiation. Although radiation should have lesser fetal effects in the third trimester, a live fetus spontaneously delivered after radiation in the third trimester has been described, demonstrating microcephaly and mental retardation [51]. Viable fetuses should be delivered by cesarean section and treatment started promptly. Ovarian transposition can be considered at the time of cesarean delivery. In women who wish to delay treatment of advanced disease for fetal indications, the use of neoadjuvant chemotherapy has recently been reported demonstrating good response rates in the two cases presented and no adverse fetal outcomes [52]. The general principles of administering chemotherapy in the gravid patient apply, and in most cases, minimal fetal effects are seen. Multidisciplinary counseling is paramount.

Newer technologies are under development that allow women a choice of fertility-sparing procedures designed to treat early stage cervical cancer. Their use following pregnancy has not been studied. Often, gravid women desire future fertility, and preservation of both ovarian function and the uterine fundus is critical to achieve this outcome. In highly select patients, delayed surgical therapy by radical trachelectomy and pelvic lymphadenectomy may be a valid option after delivery and postpartum recovery. Patients should understand the relative novelty of the procedure in the nongravid state and the lack of outcomes data in this scenario. With careful counseling, however, options for more conservative therapy may be acceptable.

## Effects of pregnancy after cervical cancer treatment

Although a diagnosis of invasive cervical cancer during pregnancy can jeopardize the life of both the mother and the fetus, the diagnosis of cervical dysplasia and early invasive cancer can have a deleterious impact on future fertility of the mother and outcomes of future fetuses. Level III data are emerging that help to define the risks of excisional therapies for dysplasia and micro-invasive cancers. A retrospective cohort study demonstrated no difference in pre-term delivery but a 1.9- and 2.7-fold increase in premature ruptured membranes in pregnancies following loop electrocautery excision procedure (LEEP) or laser conization, respectively [53]. This increase was also proportional to the amount of cervical tissue resected. Although this and other studies suggest a better pregnancy outcome with laser vaporization, this also seems to be respective of the amount of tissue destroyed [53,54]. Preterm delivery was associated with ablated cone height of 10 mm or greater [54]. A systematic review of the earlier literature also confirmed an odds ratio of 3.23 for preterm delivery following cervical conization [55]. These compelling data need to be considered when deciding cervical conization and depth of resection in women in their reproductive years.

Recent advances in surgical technique now allow opportunity for select patients with early invasive cervical cancer to maintain fertility while receiving adequate radical treatment. The procedure, known as "radical trachelectomy" with pelvic lymphadenectomy, maintains the surgical principle of removing a small central tumor (cervix) with adequate uninvolved margins (parametrium) while maintaining the uterine body for support of future pregnancies [56,57]. It can be done by a vaginal or abdominal approach [57,58]. Women desirous of future fertility who have stage IA1 lesions with lymphovascular invasion, IA2, and small IB1 squamous tumors (≤2 cm) are candidates. Few leading centers have accrued the most outcomes measures for this fertility-sparing treatment. To date, 11 (4%) of 277 reported patients have had recurrences, most outside of the immediate central pelvis [59]. Two central pelvic recurrences have been described, one with greater than 1 cm negative margins [60,61]. Seven of these 11 are dead of disease. Subsequent pregnancies see similar first-trimester loss rates (17%) as in the general population; however, second-trimester loss rates are higher (12%) [59]. Premature delivery is higher in these patients, and the permanent cerclage necessitated cesarean delivery in all. In a review by Petignat and coworkers [62], of 55 pregnancies, 22 (58%) delivered ≥36 weeks, but 15 (27%) delivered between 24 and 35 weeks gestation. Benardini and coworkers [63] studied 80 patients completing radical trachelectomy. Thirty-nine patients attempted conception with 22 pregnancies in 18 women. Eighty-two percent were viable but only 55% were delivered at term. Limited experience is available for the use of this technique in the appropriate candidate after pregnancy, but the concept is valid and should be considered in the algorithm [40]. Pregnancies after radical trachelectomy for cervical cancer are a high-risk pregnancy and should be managed immediately by a multidisciplinary team.

## Summary

Cervical cancer and dysplasia in pregnancy can be a stressful situation for both the mother and physician. Conservative management is the rule, and experts in cervical dysplasia and cancer can help to counsel the pregnant woman and carefully follow the lesions, allowing the optimal management for both the mother and the fetus. Multidisciplinary team approaches help to maximize both maternal and fetal outcomes.

## References

[1] Brown D, Berran P, Kaplan KJ, et al. Special situations: abnormal cervical cytology during pregnancy. Clin Obstet Gynecol 2005;48:178–85.

[2] Lishner M. Cancer in pregnancy. Ann Oncol 2003;14(Suppl 3):iii31–6.

[3] Nguyen C, Montz FJ, Bristow RE. Management of stage I cervical cancer in pregnancy. Obstet Gynecol Surv 2000;55:633–43.

[4] Andras EJ, Fletcher GH, Rutledge F. Radiotherapy of carcinoma of the cervix following simple hysterectomy. Am J Obstet Gynecol 1973;115:647–55.

[5] Roman LD, Morris M, Mitchell MF, et al. Prognostic factors for patients undergoing simple hysterectomy in the presence of invasive cancer of the cervix. Gynecol Oncol 1993;50: 179–84.

[6] Oduncu FS, Kimmig R, Hepp H, et al. Cancer in pregnancy: maternal-fetal conflict. J Cancer Res Clin Oncol 2003;129:133–46.

[7] Creasman WT. Cancer and pregnancy. Ann N Y Acad Sci 2001;943:281–6.

[8] Bosch FX, de Sanjose S. Human papillomavirus and cervical cancer: burden and assessment of causality. J Natl Cancer Inst Monogr 2003;31:3–13.

[9] Schiffman M, Castle PE. Human papillomavirus: epidemiology and public health. Arch Pathol Lab Med 2003;127:930–4.

[10] Tseng CJ, Liang CC, Soong YK, et al. Perinatal transmission of human papillomavirus in infants: relationship between infection rate and mode of delivery. Obstet Gynecol 1998;91:92–6.

[11] Hallden C, Majmudar B. The relationship between juvenile laryngeal papillomatosis and maternal condylomata acuminata. J Reprod Med 1986;31:804–7.

[12] Obalek S, Misiewicz J, Jablonska S, et al. Childhood condyloma acuminatum: association with genital and cutaneous human papillomaviruses. Pediatr Dermatol 1993;10:101–6.

[13] Connor JP. Noninvasive cervical cancer complicating pregnancy. Obstet Gynecol Clin North Am 1998;25:331–42.

[14] Castle PE, Wacholder S, Lorincz AT, et al. A prospective study of high-grade cervical neoplasia risk among human papillomavirus-infected women. J Natl Cancer Inst 2002;94: 1406–14.

[15] Smith EM, Ritchie JM, Yankowitz J, et al. HPV prevalence and concordance in the cervix and oral cavity of pregnant women. Infect Dis Obstet Gynecol 2004;12:45–56.

[16] Solomon D, Schiffman M, Tarone R. Comparison of three management strategies for patients with atypical squamous cells of undetermined significance: baseline results from a randomized trial. J Natl Cancer Inst 2001;93:293–9.

[17] Chan PK, Chang AR, Tam WH, et al. Prevalence and genotype distribution of cervical human papillomavirus infection: comparison between pregnant women and non-pregnant controls. J Med Virol 2002;67:583–8.

[18] Londo R, Bjelland T, Girod C, et al. Prenatal and postpartum Pap smears: do we need both? Fam Pract Res J 1994;14:359–67.

[19] Cannon JM, Blythe JG. Comparison of the Cytobrush plus plastic spatula with the Cervex Brush for obtaining endocervical cells. Obstet Gynecol 1993;82(4 Pt 1):569–72.

[20] McCord ML, Stovall TG, Meric JL, et al. Cervical cytology: a randomized comparison of four sampling methods. Am J Obstet Gynecol 1992;166(6 Pt 1):1772–7 [discussion: 1777–9].

[21] Paraiso MF, Brady K, Helmchen R, et al. Evaluation of the endocervical Cytobrush and Cervex-Brush in pregnant women. Obstet Gynecol 1994;84:539–43.

[22] Rivlin ME, Woodliff JM, Bowlin RB, et al. Comparison of cytobrush and cotton swab for Papanicolaou smears in pregnancy. J Reprod Med 1993;38:147–50.

[23] Kim JJ, Wright TC, Goldie SJ. Cost-effectiveness of alternative triage strategies for atypical squamous cells of undetermined significance. JAMA 2002;287:2382–90.

[24] Lee KR, Ashfaq R, Birdsong GG, et al. Comparison of conventional Papanicolaou smears and a fluid-based, thin-layer system for cervical cancer screening. Obstet Gynecol 1997;90: 278–84.

[25] Economos K, Perez Veridiano N, Delke I, et al. Abnormal cervical cytology in pregnancy: a 17-year experience. Obstet Gynecol 1993;81:915–8.

[26] Wright Jr TC, Cox JT, Massad LS, et al. 2001 Consensus Guidelines for the management of women with cervical cytological abnormalities. JAMA 2002;287:2120–9.

[27] Robinson WR, Luck MB, Kendall MA, et al. The predictive value of cytologic testing in women

with the human immunodeficiency virus who have low-grade squamous cervical lesions: a substudy of a randomized, phase III chemoprevention trial. Am J Obstet Gynecol 2003;188: 896–900.

[28] Hannigan EV. Cervical cancer in pregnancy. Clin Obstet Gynecol 1990;33:837–45.

[29] Ostergard DR, Nieberg RK. Evaluation of abnormal cervical cytology during pregnancy with colposcopy. Am J Obstet Gynecol 1979;134:756–8.

[30] Holowaty P, Miller AB, Rohan T, et al. Natural history of dysplasia of the uterine cervix. J Natl Cancer Inst 1999;91:252–8.

[31] Ahdoot D, Van Nostrand KM, Nguyen NJ, et al. The effect of route of delivery on regression of abnormal cervical cytologic findings in the postpartum period. Am J Obstet Gynecol 1998;178: 1116–20.

[32] Kaplan KJ, Dainty LA, Dolinsky B, et al. Prognosis and recurrence risk for patients with cervical squamous intraepithelial lesions diagnosed during pregnancy. Cancer 2004;102:228–32.

[33] Yost NP, Santoso JT, McIntire DD, et al. Postpartum regression rates of antepartum cervical intraepithelial neoplasia II and III lesions. Obstet Gynecol 1999;93:359–62.

[34] Paraskevaidis E, Koliopoulos G, Kalantaridou S, et al. Management and evolution of cervical intraepithelial neoplasia during pregnancy and postpartum. Eur J Obstet Gynecol Reprod Biol 2002;104:67–9.

[35] Siddiqui G, Kurzel RB, Lampley EC, et al. Cervical dysplasia in pregnancy: progression versus regression post-partum. Int J Fertil Womens Med 2001;46:278–80.

[36] Goldberg GL, Altaras MM, Block B. Cone cerclage in pregnancy. Obstet Gynecol 1991;77: 315–7.

[37] Sood AK, Sorosky JI. Invasive cervical cancer complicating pregnancy: how to manage the dilemma. Obstet Gynecol Clin North Am 1998;25:343–52.

[38] Sorosky JI. Cervical cancer complicating pregnancy: two patients with three clinical objectives. Obstet Gynecol 2004;104(5 Pt 2):1127–8.

[39] Sorosky JI, Squatrito R, Ndubisi BU, et al. Stage I squamous cell cervical carcinoma in pregnancy: planned delay in therapy awaiting fetal maturity. Gynecol Oncol 1995;59:207–10.

[40] Ben-Arie A, Levy R, Lavie O, et al. Conservative treatment of stage IA2 squamous cell carcinoma of the cervix during pregnancy. Obstet Gynecol 2004;104(5 Pt 2):1129–31.

[41] Sood AK, Sorosky JI, Krogman S, et al. Surgical management of cervical cancer complicating pregnancy: a case-control study. Gynecol Oncol 1996;63:294–8.

[42] Takushi M, Moromizato H, Sakumoto K, et al. Management of invasive carcinoma of the uterine cervix associated with pregnancy: outcome of intentional delay in treatment. Gynecol Oncol 2002;87:185–9.

[43] Burghardt E, Ostor A, Fox H. The new FIGO definition of cervical cancer stage IA: a critique. Gynecol Oncol 1997;65:1–5.

[44] Goldman NA, Goldberg GL. Late recurrence of squamous cell cervical cancer in an episiotomy site after vaginal delivery. Obstet Gynecol 2003;101(5 Pt 2):1127–9.

[45] Sood AK, Sorosky JI, Mayr N, et al. Cervical cancer diagnosed shortly after pregnancy: prognostic variables and delivery routes. Obstet Gynecol 2000;95(6 Pt 1):832–8.

[46] Monk BJ, Montz FJ. Invasive cervical cancer complicating intrauterine pregnancy: treatment with radical hysterectomy. Obstet Gynecol 1992;80:199–203.

[47] Yessaian A, Magistris A, Burger RA, et al. Radical hysterectomy followed by tailored postoperative therapy in the treatment of stage IB2 cervical cancer: feasibility and indications for adjuvant therapy. Gynecol Oncol 2004;94:61–6.

[48] Sood AK, Sorosky JI, Mayr N, et al. Radiotherapeutic management of cervical carcinoma that complicates pregnancy. Cancer 1997;80:1073–8.

[49] Sklar C. Maintenance of ovarian function and risk of premature menopause related to cancer treatment. J Natl Cancer Inst Monogr 2005;34:25–7.

[50] Fielding JR. MR imaging of the female pelvis. Radiol Clin North Am 2003;41:179–92.

[51] Gustavson KH, Jagell S, Blomquist HK, et al. Microcephaly, mental retardation and chromosomal aberrations in a girl following radiation therapy during late fetal life. Acta Radiol Oncol 1981;20:209–12.

[52] Tewari K, Cappuccini F, Gambino A, et al. Neoadjuvant chemotherapy in the treatment of locally advanced cervical carcinoma in pregnancy: a report of two cases and review of issues specific to the management of cervical carcinoma in pregnancy including planned delay of therapy. Cancer 1998;82:1529–34.

[53] Sadler L, Saftlas A, Wang W, et al. Treatment for cervical intraepithelial neoplasia and risk of preterm delivery. JAMA 2004;291:2100–6.

[54] Raio L, Ghezzi F, Di Naro E, et al. Duration of pregnancy after carbon dioxide laser conization of the cervix: influence of cone height. Obstet Gynecol 1997;90:978–82.

[55] Kristensen J, Langhoff-Roos J, Wittrup M, et al. Cervical conization and preterm delivery/low birth weight: a systematic review of the literature. Acta Obstet Gynecol Scand 1993;72:640–4.

[56] Shepherd JH, Crawford RA, Oram DH. Radical trachelectomy: a way to preserve fertility in the treatment of early cervical cancer. Br J Obstet Gynaecol 1998;105:912–6.

[57] Smith JR, Boyle DC, Corless DJ, et al. Abdominal radical trachelectomy: a new surgical technique for the conservative management of cervical carcinoma. Br J Obstet Gynaecol 1997;104:1196–200.

[58] Dargent D, Martin X, Sacchetoni A, et al. Laparoscopic vaginal radical trachelectomy: a treatment to preserve the fertility of cervical carcinoma patients. Cancer 2000;88:1877–82.

[59] Gershenson DM. Fertility-sparing surgery for malignancies in women. J Natl Cancer Inst Monogr 2005;34:43–7.

[60] Bali A, Weekes A, Van Trappen P, et al. Central pelvic recurrence 7 years after radical vaginal trachelectomy. Gynecol Oncol 2005;96:854–6.

[61] Del Priore G, Ungar L, Richard Smith J, et al. Regarding "First case of a centropelvic recurrence after radical trachelectomy: literature review and implications for the preoperative selection of patients," (92:1002–5) by Morice et al. Gynecol Oncol 2004;95:414 [author reply: 414–6].

[62] Petignat P, Stan C, Megevand E, et al. Pregnancy after trachelectomy: a high-risk condition of preterm delivery. Report of a case and review of the literature. Gynecol Oncol 2004;94:575–7.

[63] Bernardini M, Barrett J, Seaward G, et al. Pregnancy outcomes in patients after radical trachelectomy. Am J Obstet Gynecol 2003;189:1378–82.

OBSTETRICS AND
GYNECOLOGY
CLINICS
OF NORTH AMERICA

Obstet Gynecol Clin N Am
32 (2005) 547–558

# Breast Cancer and Pregnancy

## Kimberly K. Leslie, MD[a],*, Carol A. Lange, Phd[b]

[a]Division of Maternal-Fetal Medicine, Department of Obstetrics and Gynecology,
University of New Mexico Health Sciences Center, 2211 Lomas Boulevard NE, ACC-4,
Albuquerque, NM 87131, USA
[b]Departments of Medicine and Pharmacology, University of Minnesota, 425 East River Road,
Suite 460 C, Minneapolis, MN 55455, USA

The lifetime probability of developing breast cancer, assuming a life span of 85 years, was reported to be 13% for white women and 9% for black women as of 1993 [1]; it is likely that the incidence has continued to increase over the past decade. Although most women who have breast cancer are postmenopausal, the number of cases in younger women seems to be disproportionately on the rise. Younger women have the worst survival outcomes when matched with similarly staged older women. They more often have positive lymph nodes, larger tumors, negative steroid hormone receptors, a higher S-phase fraction (the percent of cells in the DNA synthesis stage of the cell cycle), *BRCA1* and *BRCA2* mutations [2], and downregulation or mutation of the tumor suppressor gene p53 [3]. The worse outcome for younger patients is consistent with the fact that more of the cases are familial; many cases of breast cancer in younger women also are associated with pregnancy.

Breast cancer is considered to be associated with pregnancy if the diagnosis is made during a pregnancy or within 1 year of delivery [4]. Approximately 1 in 3000 to 10,000 women are diagnosed with a malignant breast tumor that is associated with a pregnancy [5–8]. From 32 series of the total number of women with breast cancer, 0.2% to 3.8% of the patients had a pregnancy-associated tumor [9]. It is estimated that 10 to 39 women per 100,000 live births are diagnosed with breast cancer during pregnancy [10], and a transient increase in breast cancer risk has been documented immediately after delivery [11]. For premenopausal women, it is striking that one in three to four breast cancers is

---

* Corresponding author.
*E-mail address:* kleslie@salud.unm.edu (K.K. Leslie).

associated with pregnancy according to the precise definition [12,13]. Given the potentially prolonged occult growth period of breast tumors, it is likely that many more cancers are present during and influenced by a preceding pregnancy, perhaps years before the diagnosis is actually made. Pregnancy association is a risk factor because the normal physiologic breast changes of pregnancy may mask a developing malignant mass and result in a significant delay in diagnosis [14]. The elevated levels of hormones in pregnancy, principally estrogen and progesterone, may have a stimulatory effect on breast cancer growth, and the pregnancy itself and concerns for fetal well-being may impact the treatment options available for the mother. Although pregnancy and lactation are reported to decrease the overall risk of breast cancer in older women [15–18], for individuals younger than age 35 who are diagnosed with breast cancer, the association with pregnancy predicts a worse outcome. For example, Largent and colleagues [19] described a population case case study of 254 women diagnosed with invasive breast cancer younger than age 35. Compared with nulliparous women, women with three or more births were more likely to be diagnosed with a nonlocalized tumor, a poor prognostic finding. The researchers also found that women with two or more full-term pregnancies were more likely to die from their disease compared with women with one or no term pregnancy. These data seem to indicate that among younger women, tumors associated with pregnancy are more aggressive and more difficult to treat. In particular, women who have had multiple pregnancies during the period of tumorigenesis are at risk for worse outcomes.

In the case of women who carry mutations in the tumor suppressor genes *BRCA1* or *BRCA2*, the lifetime risk for breast cancer is 80%. [20,21]. Recent reports have addressed the effect of pregnancy on lifetime risk for breast cancer in this population. The effect of parity seems to be different depending on whether the patient carries a mutation in *BRCA1* or *BRCA2*. From a study of 1260 pairs of women with known mutations compared with unaffected controls, women who carried *BRCA1* mutations and had four or more births had a 38% reduction in breast cancer risk compared with nulliparous women with the same mutation, which indicated a modest protective effect [2]. For women with *BRCA2* mutations, increasing parity was associated with a significant increase in the risk of breast cancer before age 50, and this increase was greatest in the 2-year period after a pregnancy [2]. The effect of pregnancy on breast cancer risk may vary depending on the genomic mutations and variants present in an individual or population.

**Physiology and anatomy**

The breast undergoes remarkable epithelial cell hypertrophy during pregnancy. The breast is composed of two major cell populations: epithelial and mesenchymal. The epithelial cells line the ducts, whereas the mesenchymal cells make up the stroma. Beginning early in the course of pregnancy and continuing throughout gestation, the epithelial cells undergo rapid proliferation, which alters the ratio of epithelial to mesenchymal cells [22]. The lymphatics and blood vessels also significantly increase in size and number. Breast hypertrophy is related to hormonal changes during pregnancy with a rise in estradiol, estrone, estriol, progesterone, cortisol, insulin, and prolactin. Each of these hormones is involved in the increase in breast tissue and the maturation of the ducts and lobules that are required for lactation. The circulating progesterone concentration increases more than 1000-fold compared with the nonpregnant levels, estrogens increase more than 100-fold, corticosteroids increase between two- and threefold, and insulin and prolactin are also significantly elevated [23].

## Receptors and mechanisms of tumorigenesis

Steroid hormones, such as estrogen and progesterone, act through intracellular transcription factors called steroid receptors. These factors bind to the promoters of hormone-responsive genes and control the production of mRNA and the encoded proteins. Receptors for estrogen and progesterone are typically abundant in breast cancers and are a sign of cellular differentiation. Tumors with estrogen and progesterone have a better prognosis than those without receptors. Compared with breast cancers that are not associated with pregnancy, estrogen levels in pregnancy-associated tumors are often low or absent, which is a poor prognostic sign [24].

Estrogen and progesterone clearly play a vital role in mammary gland development. Studies that used estrogen and progesterone knock-out mice demonstrated that estrogen is required for the growth and elongation of mammary ductal structures [25], whereas progesterone is required for the formation and growth of the lobular alveoli (milk-producing glands) located at the ends of ducts [26,27]. Remarkably, steroid hormone receptor–positive cells account for only 10% to 20% of the luminal epithelial cells that line the ducts and lobular alveoli in the adult resting (nonpregnant) premenopausal breast [28]. In the normal breast, these cells do not divide but are often located adjacent to dividing cells that are estrogen/progesterone negative. Progesterone-positive epithelial cells are believed to express and secrete locally acting growth factors (Wnts, insulin-like growth factor-II), which then stimulate the proliferation of adjacent progesterone-negative epithelial cells [29,30]. Interactions between proliferating (progesterone-negative) and nonproliferating (progesterone-positive) epithelial cells with the surrounding stromal cells are also important for the maintenance of the normal breast. An early event in breast cancer development seems to be the disruption of normal cell-cell communication and a switch to autocrine mechanisms of proliferation within the steroid hormone receptor–positive population. This receptor-positive cell population comprises 80% of breast cancers, and the earliest breast cancer lesions (breast carcinoma in situ) most often express steroid hormone receptors, unlike nonmalignant breast tissue [31,32].

Estrogen- and progesterone-positive breast cancer cells are stimulated to proliferate in response to estrogens, and antiestrogen and aromatase inhibitor therapies are based on this property of steroid hormone-sensitive breast cancers. As tumors progress, however, they often lose their sensitivity to endocrine-based treatments (regardless of receptor status) and resume growth in the presence of estrogen-blocking agents or inhibitors of local estrogen production. Approximately 60% to 70% of advanced breast cancers are steroid hormone resistant, whereas most retain steroid hormone receptor expression [33]. The mechanisms of breast cancer progression from steroid hormone–sensitive to steroid hormone–resistant phenotypes are complex. A key event seems to be upregulation of transmembrane tyrosine kinase growth factor receptors, however. For example, progestins upregulate the expression of epidermal growth factor receptor family members, including erbB2 [34,35]. Insulin-like growth factor-1 receptors are also overexpressed in most breast cancer cells [36,37]. Steroid hormones (via the transcriptional activities of estrogen and progesterone) also regulate the expression of proteins (IRS-1, IRS-2) that are required signaling components in the insulin-like growth factor-I pathway, including the insulin-like growth factor-IR [36]. Steroid hormones, via the action of their nuclear receptors, mediate changes in gene expression that, in turn, make breast epithelial cells competent to receive signals from systemic or locally acting peptide growth factors. This process is important for normal breast development. During breast cancer progression, however, increased sensitivity of breast cancer cells to growth factor mitogens is likely mediated by similar mechanisms, and these two classes of hormones (ie, steroid hormones and peptide growth factors) often synergize to effect changes in gene expression that may contribute to increased cell growth, proliferation, and survival of breast tumor cells.

Estrogen and progesterone exist on DNA in a complex with other proteins that regulate receptor transcriptional activity positively (coactivators) or negatively (co-repressors). Another level of control occurs via protein phosphorylation. The receptors and the comodulators are heavily phosphorylated and activated in response to stimulation by mitogenic (ie, peptide growth factor) signaling pathways and protein kinases in breast cancer cells. Steroid receptor or co-regulator phosphorylation has been studied extensively as a mechanism of breast cancer cell escape from steroid hormone regulation. For example, phosphorylation of estrogen, progesterone, or their transcriptional coactivators (SRC-1, SRC-3/AIB1) increases transcriptional activity on diverse promoters. This process usually occurs only in response to or in the presence of hormone (ligand) and is regulated; however, unregulated and constitutive signaling from mitogenic pathways can mediate transcriptional activation of these receptors in the absence of steroid hormones and during hormone ablation [38–41]. In the face of heightened protein kinase activities commonly associated with breast cancer progression, steroid hormone receptors become hyperactive or hypersensitive [42]. Phosphorylation events can alter steroid hormone receptor subcellular location and influence receptor levels by increasing the rate of receptor turnover via protein degradative pathways [43]. Hyperactive receptors are predicted to turn over rapidly

[40,44,45]. Breast cancers (particularly in the setting of pregnancy) may seem to be estrogen/progesterone negative but instead may contain low levels of highly active receptors. Receptor phosphorylation also alters promoter selectivity; different phospho-species of the same steroid hormone receptor regulate different gene subsets [46,47]. Such altered genetic programming is believed to contribute to breast cancer progression.

In addition to stimulation of steroid hormone receptor protein loss by increased turnover, growth factor signaling ultimately induces the downregulation of estrogen and progesterone mRNAs at the level of gene regulation/transcription [48,49]. Breast cancers with high constitutive expression of epidermal growth factor receptor or ErbB2 often display loss or absence of steroid hormone receptors. Estrogen and highly activated epidermal growth factor receptor/Ras/Raf do not seem to coexist in the same cells within estrogen-positive tumors, and inhibition of epidermal growth factor receptor signaling can restore estrogen expression, which indicates that changes that occur during breast tumor progression may be reversible [49]. Breast tumors tend to progress from a state of hormone sensitivity to hormone hypersensitivity and finally toward hormone insensitivity.

The responsiveness of breast cancer cells to estrogens and progestins depends highly on the presence of additional growth factors and cytokines and the relative concentrations of steroid hormone receptors and their ligands. Although epidermal growth factor can potentiate progesterone-dependent breast cancer cell growth [50,51], progestins can induce cell death via apoptosis in the presence of selected cytokines, including tumor necrosis factor-alpha, interleukin-beta, and interferon-gamma [52]. High ($10^{-4}$M) but not low ($10^{-10}$M) concentrations of progesterone induce apoptotic cell death and loss of BRCA1 and cyclin A in breast cancer cells [53]. These effects may be especially relevant to pregnancy, during which estrogen and progesterone levels are 100-fold and 1000-fold higher, respectively, relative to the nonpregnant state. Under these conditions, receptors are predicted to be saturated, functionally active, and rapidly turning over (ie, apparent low abundance). Elimination of progesterone-positive breast epithelial cells via apoptosis under conditions of high circulating progesterone concentrations may explain partly the protection from breast cancer development conferred by early pregnancy and why termination of pregnancy does not significantly improve the outcome of established breast cancers (see later discussion).

**Diagnosis**

Epithelial cell hypertrophy and resultant breast enlargement make the diagnosis of breast cancer difficult during pregnancy, and the best opportunity to obtain an adequate breast examination by palpation is early in the first trimester. Thereafter, a dominant mass is less likely to be palpable. If a mass is suspected, however, an evaluation is indicated immediately; it is not appropriate to wait until after delivery. Because of the difficulties encountered in physical examination and radiologic assessment during pregnancy, the diagnosis of breast cancer is delayed from the time of symptom onset in pregnancy from 9 to 15 months. The average size at diagnosis is 3.5 cm for pregnancy-associated tumors compared with less than 2 cm for tumors diagnosed remote from pregnancy.

The most common symptoms experienced by women with breast cancer during pregnancy are a new dominant mass and nipple discharge. In general, patients with a dominant mass or abnormal nipple discharge during pregnancy should have the same diagnostic evaluation as their nonpregnant counterparts. Many pregnant women experience nipple discharge during pregnancy; however, the discharge is usually clear or slightly milky and arises from multiple ducts. For purposes of discussion, abnormal nipple discharge should be considered to be present if only one duct is involved or if the discharge is bloody or purulent.

Mammography, the most important diagnostic test used in the evaluation of a breast mass, may be unreliable because of the density of the pregnant breast. In pregnancy, mammography is acceptable from the standpoint of radiation exposure to the fetus; however, the test is likely to be nondiagnostic because of the density of the pregnant breast and cannot be relied on to rule out malignancy. In a small study of eight pregnant women with breast cancer who underwent mammograms, six of the eight studies were negative [54]. Ultrasonography can be used to distinguish fluid-filled cysts from solid masses. If cystic, aspiration of the fluid should be performed and the fluid should be sent for cytologic evaluation if it is bloody. If the fluid is clear, many practitioners believe that cytologic evaluation is not necessary; however, the mass should be followed to ensure that fluid does not reaccumulate. Fine-needle aspiration of a solid mass is less accurate in pregnancy because of the normal hyperplastic epithelial changes and must be interpreted by an experienced pathologist. Not infrequently, fine-needle aspirations of breast masses during pregnancy are nondiagnostic and may be labeled falsely as malignant [55]. In general, if a solid mass is found, surgical excision is the standard practice and usually can be performed under local anesthesia (although general anesthesia is certainly not contraindicated in pregnancy) [23]. Excisional biopsies may be complicated by infection, hematomas, and milk fistulas. Prophylactic antibiotics should be given and patients should consider ceasing lactation if the biopsy is performed in the postpartum period. Byrd and colleagues [56] reported that of 134 biopsies performed during pregnancy or lactation, 29 proved to be cancer.

## Staging

Once carcinoma of the breast is diagnosed, staging must be performed to rule out metastatic disease. This step is important because an operative cure is unlikely if metastatic disease is present. In addition to a complete history and a detailed physical examination, laboratory tests should be ordered, such as a complete blood count and a biochemical analysis, including liver function tests. Radiologic tests are also indicated, and most are within the acceptable range with respect to radiation exposure to the fetus, which should be limited to no more than 5 cGy (mrad) according to the American Academy of Pediatrics in an opinion rendered in 1978. Fortunately, most screening tests result in far lower exposures. For example, a chest radiograph results in approximately 0.008 cGy when abdominal shielding is used, and a chest radiograph is indicated in the staging evaluation of all patients. Nuclear magnetic resonance (NMR) is accepted as safe in pregnancy and may be preferable to CT scans; in general, however, CT scans are not contraindicated in pregnancy. For clinical stage I and II disease, bone scans are not indicated unless a patient has symptoms or serum chemistries that suggest bone involvement. For clinical stage III disease, however, a modified bone scan using maternal hydration reported by Baker and colleagues [57] reduces the fetal radiation exposure to an acceptable 76 mrem resulting from the isotope $^{99m}$Tc. Unless a patient has central nervous system symptoms, a brain scan is rarely performed.

## Treatment

The general treatment approach is the same for the pregnant state as for the nonpregnant state. For disease that is clinically nonmetastatic based on the staging evaluation, however, a modified radical mastectomy is still the standard for breast cancers associated with pregnancy, although recent reports of conservative surgical procedures, including lumpectomy with node biopsies, have appeared in the literature [58]. Lumpectomy with radiotherapy to follow has been reported to result in unacceptably high radiation doses to the fetus. The fetal radiation dose has been reported to be 0.2% to 2% of the maternal dose [59]. For the standard breast radiotherapy course of 5000 cGy, most clinicians anticipate 10 cGy in early pregnancy and 200 cGy in late pregnancy. Because these levels are above the recommended pregnancy limit of safety (5 cGy), breast conservation and radiotherapy is typically not recommended in pregnancy. The risk of radiation depends on the trimester of exposure, however. From the day of conception to day 10 (the preimplantation period), the outcome that results from a significant radiation exposure is either normal or fetal death. This is a general rule because the cells of the preimplantation conceptus are pluripotent: if a small proportion of the cells are damaged, others can multiply and take their place. If too many cells die, however, the conceptus dies. From day 10 to week 8 (the period of organogenesis), severe malformations are possible, especially if the exposure is more than 5 cGy. From 8 weeks to term (the fetal period), malformations are less likely, but microcephaly and intrauterine growth restriction may occur. The possibility of childhood cancers is also slightly increased with a relative risk of 1.5 [60], and genetic effects in subsequent generations are possible if gamete DNA is damaged [61]. It should be noted that recent opinions may be softening on the use of radiotherapy during pregnancy. The reader is referred to a review by Kal and Struikmans [62], which suggests that radiotherapy during pregnancy may not be contraindicated provided that appropriate shielding is in place.

For surgery, general anesthesia is indicated. Antacids should be given to raise the gastric pH. This precaution is required because of the increased risk of aspiration with pregnancy. Prolonged preoxygenation before endotracheal intubation should be undertaken, and intraoperative fetal monitoring should be considered during the procedure so that anesthesia can be adjusted to avoid fetal hypoxia. The patient also should undergo fetal and uterine monitoring in the early postoperative period to rule out fetal distress and preterm labor. Postoperative tocolysis should be instituted if necessary.

For stage II or greater disease, chemotherapy is the standard of care. Chemotherapy with a combination of cyclophosphamide, adriamycin, and 5-fluorouracil versus cyclophosphamide alone is commonly used. Other regimens, including those with paclitaxel, have been reported [63–65]. Most clinicians avoid the folate inhibitor methotrexate during pregnancy. Malformation rates of 17% to 25% have been reported with methotrexate compared with 6% with cyclophosphamide alone [66]. These numbers compare with the baseline malformation rate of 3% in the general population. In addition to malformations, fetal growth abnormalities may result from chemotherapy. According to one report, nearly 40% of infants exposed to chemotherapy in utero were growth restricted [67], although more recent studies indicate that the risk for intrauterine growth restriction may be less than previously reported [63,64,68].

The role of therapeutic abortion in the management of breast cancer in pregnancy has been debated. An evolution in thinking has occurred in the past three decades. It is clear that there is no benefit to the mother for performing a therapeutic abortion. Abortion may be indicated if significant fetal effects as a consequence of therapy are expected, however (ie, the diagnosis is made in early pregnancy). Regarding the controversy as to whether induced or spontaneous abortion increases the risk of developing breast cancer later in life, a thorough review of the literature and reanalysis indicate that pregnancies that end in a spontaneous or induced abortion do not increase a woman's risk of developing breast cancer [69].

## Prognosis

Stage for stage, the outcome is the same [70–72]; however, pregnant women present with more advanced disease: 28% in stage I, 30% in stage II, and 47% in stage III and IV [23]. Lymph node metastasis is common and is present in 65% of patients with pregnancy-associated breast cancer. The overall survival rate is 70% [73]. The 5-year survival rate for patients with negative nodes in pregnancy is 82%, which is identical to patients who are not pregnant [14]. A reassuring fact is that a subsequent pregnancy does not result in a poorer outcome for women who have been treated for breast cancer [9,74]. It is prudent wait 2 to 5 years after diagnosis and treatment, however, to ensure that a recurrence is not eminent [4].

## References

[1] Feuer EJ, Wun LM, Boring CC, et al. The lifetime risk of developing breast cancer. J Natl Cancer Inst 1993;85(11):892–7.

[2] Cullinane CA, Lubinski J, Neuhausen SL, et al. Effect of pregnancy as a risk factor for breast cancer in BRCA1/BRCA2 mutation carriers. Int J Cancer 2005;117(6):988–91.

[3] Albain KS, Allred DC, Clark GM. Breast cancer outcome and predictors of outcome: are there age differentials? J Natl Cancer Inst Monogr 1994;16:35–42.

[4] Petrek JA. Breast cancer and pregnancy. J Natl Cancer Inst Monogr 1994;16:113–21.

[5] White TT. Carcinoma of the breast and pregnancy: analysis of 920 cases collected from the literature and 22 new cases. Ann Surg 1954;139(1):9–18.

[6] White TT. Prognosis of breast cancer for pregnant and nursing women: analysis of 1,413 cases. Surg Gynecol Obstet 1955;100(6):661–6.

[7] Peete Jr CH, Huneycutt Jr HC, Cherny WB. Cancer of the breast in pregnancy. N C Med J 1966; 27(11):514–20.

[8] Anderson JM. Mammary cancers and pregnancy. BMJ 1979;1(6171):1124–7.

[9] Wallack MK, Wolf Jr JA, Bedwinek J, et al. Gestational carcinoma of the female breast. Curr Probl Cancer 1983;7(9):1–58.

[10] Gemignani ML, Petrek JA. Pregnancy-associated breast cancer: diagnosis and treatment. Breast J 2000;6(1):68–73.

[11] Liu Q, Wuu J, Lambe M, et al. Transient increase in breast cancer risk after giving birth: postpartum period with the highest risk (Sweden). Cancer Causes Control 2002;13(4):299–305.

[12] Horsley III JS, Alrich EM, Wright CB. Carcinoma of the breast in women 35 years of age or younger. Ann Surg 1969;169(6):839–43.

[13] Finn WF. Pregnancy complicated by cancer. Bull Jersey City Margaret Hague Mat Hosp 1952; 5(255):2–6.

[14] Petrek JA, Dukoff R, Rogatko A. Prognosis of pregnancy-associated breast cancer. Cancer 1991;67(4):869–72.

[15] Albrektsen G, Heuch I, Kvale G. The short-term and long-term effect of a pregnancy on breast cancer risk: a prospective study of 802,457 parous Norwegian women. Br J Cancer 1995; 72(2):480–4.

[16] Greenlee RT, Murray T, Bolden S, et al. Cancer statistics, 2000. CA Cancer J Clin 2000;50(1): 7–33.

[17] MacMahon B, Cole P, Lin TM, et al. Age at first birth and breast cancer risk. Bull World Health Organ 1970;43(2):209–21.

[18] Lambe M, Hsieh CC, Chan HW, et al. Parity, age at first and last birth, and risk of breast cancer: a population-based study in Sweden. Breast Cancer Res Treat 1996;38(3):305–11.

[19] Largent JA, Ziogas A, Anton-Culver H. Effect of reproductive factors on stage, grade and hormone receptor status in early-onset breast cancer. Breast Cancer Res 2005;7(4):R541–54.

[20] Ford D, Easton DF, Stratton M, et al. Genetic heterogeneity and penetrance analysis of the BRCA1 and BRCA2 genes in breast cancer families: the Breast Cancer Linkage Consortium. Am J Hum Genet 1998;62(3):676–89.

[21] Antoniou A, Pharoah PD, Narod S, et al. Average risks of breast and ovarian cancer associated with BRCA1 or BRCA2 mutations detected in case series unselected for family history: a combined analysis of 22 studies. Am J Hum Genet 2003;72(5):1117–30.

[22] Canter JW, Oliver GC, Zaloudek CJ. Surgical diseases of the breast during pregnancy. Clin Obstet Gynecol 1983;26(4):853–64.

[23]  Fiorica JV. Special problems: breast cancer and pregnancy. Obstet Gynecol Clin North Am 1994; 21(4):721–32.

[24]  Hubay CA, Barry FM, Marr CC. Pregnancy and breast cancer. Surg Clin North Am 1978;58(4): 819–31.

[25]  Korach KS. Insights from the study of animals lacking functional estrogen receptor. Science 1994;266(5190):1524–7.

[26]  Conneely OM, Mulac-Jericevic B, Lydon JP, et al. Reproductive functions of the progesterone receptor isoforms: lessons from knock-out mice. Mol Cell Endocrinol 2001;179(1–2): 97–103.

[27]  Lydon JP, DeMayo FJ, Conneely OM, et al. Reproductive phenotypes of the progesterone receptor null mutant mouse. J Steroid Biochem Mol Biol 1996;56(1–6 Spec No):67–77.

[28]  Clarke RB, Anderson E, Howell A, et al. Regulation of human breast epithelial stem cells. Cell Prolif 2003;36(Suppl 1):45–58.

[29]  Robinson GW, Hennighausen L, Johnson PF. Side-branching in the mammary gland: the progesterone-Wnt connection. Genes Dev 2000;14(8):889–94.

[30]  Robinson GW, Johnson PF, Hennighausen L, et al. The C/EBPbeta transcription factor regulates epithelial cell proliferation and differentiation in the mammary gland. Genes Dev 1998;12(12): 1907–16.

[31]  Clark GM, Wenger CR, Beardslee S, et al. How to integrate steroid hormone receptor, flow cytometric, and other prognostic information in regard to primary breast cancer. Cancer 1993; 71(6 Suppl):2157–62.

[32]  Osborne CK, Schiff R. Estrogen-receptor biology: continuing progress and therapeutic implications. J Clin Oncol 2005;23(8):1616–22.

[33]  Duffy MJ. Predictive markers in breast and other cancers: a review. Clin Chem 2005;51(3): 494–503.

[34]  Lange CA, Richer JK, Shen T, et al. Convergence of progesterone and epidermal growth factor signaling in breast cancer: potentiation of mitogen-activated protein kinase pathways. J Biol Chem 1998;273(47):31308–16.

[35]  Lange CA, Richer JK, Horwitz KB. Hypothesis: progesterone primes breast cancer cells for cross-talk with proliferative or antiproliferative signals. Mol Endocrinol 1999;13(6):829–36.

[36]  Surmacz E, Bartucci M. Role of estrogen receptor alpha in modulating IGF-I receptor signaling and function in breast cancer. J Exp Clin Cancer Res 2004;23(3):385–94.

[37]  Thorne C, Lee AV. Cross talk between estrogen receptor and IGF signaling in normal mammary gland development and breast cancer. Breast Dis 2003;17:105–14.

[38]  Narayanan R, Adigun AA, Edwards DP, et al. Cyclin-dependent kinase activity is required for progesterone receptor function: novel role for cyclin A/Cdk2 as a progesterone receptor coactivator. Mol Cell Biol 2005;25(1):264–77.

[39]  Font de Mora J, Brown M. AIB1 is a conduit for kinase-mediated growth factor signaling to the estrogen receptor. Mol Cell Biol 2000;20(14):5041–7.

[40]  Shen T, Horwitz KB, Lange CA. Transcriptional hyperactivity of human progesterone receptors is coupled to their ligand-dependent down-regulation by mitogen-activated protein kinase-dependent phosphorylation of serine 294. Mol Cell Biol 2001;21(18):6122–31.

[41]  Pierson-Mullany LK, Lange CA. Phosphorylation of progesterone receptor serine 400 mediates ligand-independent transcriptional activity in response to activation of cyclin-dependent protein kinase 2. Mol Cell Biol 2004;24(24):10542–57.

[42]  Qiu M, Lange CA. MAP kinases couple multiple functions of human progesterone receptors: degradation, transcriptional synergy, and nuclear association. J Steroid Biochem Mol Biol 2003; 85(2–5):147–57.

[43]  Qiu M, Olsen A, Faivre E, et al. Mitogen-activated protein kinase regulates nuclear association of human progesterone receptors. Mol Endocrinol 2003;17(4):628–42.

[44]  Dace A, Zhao L, Park KS, et al. Hormone binding induces rapid proteasome-mediated degradation of thyroid hormone receptors. Proc Natl Acad Sci U S A 2000;97(16):8985–90.

[45]  Nawaz Z, O'Malley BW. Urban renewal in the nucleus: is protein turnover by proteasomes

absolutely required for nuclear receptor-regulated transcription? Mol Endocrinol 2004;18(3): 493–9.

[46] Cidlowski JA, Richon V. Evidence for microheterogeneity in the structure of human glucocorticoid receptors. Endocrinology 1984;115(4):1588–97.

[47] Webster JC, Jewell CM, Bodwell JE, et al. Mouse glucocorticoid receptor phosphorylation status influences multiple functions of the receptor protein. J Biol Chem 1997;272(14): 9287–93.

[48] Cui X, Zhang P, Deng W, et al. Insulin-like growth factor-I inhibits progesterone receptor expression in breast cancer cells via the phosphatidylinositol 3-kinase/Akt/mammalian target of rapamycin pathway: progesterone receptor as a potential indicator of growth factor activity in breast cancer. Mol Endocrinol 2003;17(4):575–88.

[49] Oh AS, Lorant LA, Holloway JN, et al. Hyperactivation of MAPK induces loss of ERalpha expression in breast cancer cells. Mol Endocrinol 2001;15(8):1344–59.

[50] Skildum A, Faivre E, Lange CA. Progesterone receptors induce cell cycle progression via activation of mitogen-activated protein kinases. Mol Endocrinol 2005;19(2):327–39.

[51] Groshong SD, Owen GI, Grimison B, et al. Biphasic regulation of breast cancer cell growth by progesterone: role of the cyclin-dependent kinase inhibitors, p21 and p27(Kip1). Mol Endocrinol 1997;11(11):1593–607.

[52] Bentrari F, Arnould L, Jackson AP, et al. Progesterone enhances cytokine-stimulated nitric oxide synthase II expression and cell death in human breast cancer cells. Lab Invest 2005;85(5): 624–32.

[53] Ansquer Y, Legrand A, Bringuier AF, et al. Progesterone induces BRCA1 mRNA decrease, cell cycle alterations and apoptosis in the MCF7 breast cancer cell line. Anticancer Res 2005;25(1A): 243–8.

[54] Max MH, Klamer TW. Pregnancy and breast cancer. South Med J 1983;76(9):1088–90.

[55] Finley JL, Silverman JF, Lannin DR. Fine-needle aspiration cytology of breast masses in pregnant and lactating women. Diagn Cytopathol 1989;5(3):255–9.

[56] Byrd Jr BF, Bayer DS, Robertson JC, et al. Treatment of breast tumors associated with pregnancy and lactation. Ann Surg 1962;155:940–7.

[57] Baker J, Ali A, Groch MW, et al. Bone scanning in pregnant patients with breast carcinoma. Clin Nucl Med 1987;12(7):519–24.

[58] Gentilini O, Masullo M, Rotmensz N, et al. Breast cancer diagnosed during pregnancy and lactation: biological features and treatment options. Eur J Surg Oncol 2005;31(3):232–6.

[59] National Council on Radiation and Measurements. Basic radiation protection criteria, Chapter 8. Dose limiting recommendations and guidance for special cases. Published in Washington, DC. p. 92–3.

[60] Donegan WL. Breast cancer and pregnancy. Obstet Gynecol 1977;50(2):244–52.

[61] International Commission on Radiological Protection and International Commission on Radiological Units and Measurements. Exposure of man to ionizing radiation arising from medical procedures: an enquiry into methods of evaluation. Phys Med Biol 1957;2(2):107–51.

[62] Kal HB, Struikmans H. Radiotherapy during pregnancy: fact and fiction. Lancet Oncol 2005; 6(5):328–33.

[63] Ring AE, Smith IE, Jones A, et al. Chemotherapy for breast cancer during pregnancy: an 18-year experience from five London teaching hospitals. J Clin Oncol 2005;23(18):4192–7.

[64] Mathelin C, Annane K, Liegeois P, et al. Chemotherapy for breast cancer during pregnancy. Eur J Obstet Gynecol Reprod Biol 2005; Epub ahead of print. In press.

[65] Gadducci A, Cosio S, Fanucchi A, et al. Chemotherapy with epirubicin and paclitaxel for breast cancer during pregnancy: case report and review of the literature. Anticancer Res 2003;23(6D): 5225–9.

[66] Doll DC, Ringenberg QS, Yarbro JW. Management of cancer during pregnancy. Arch Intern Med 1988;148(9):2058–64.

[67] Sweet Jr DL, Kinzie J. Consequences of radiotherapy and antineoplastic therapy for the fetus. J Reprod Med 1976;17(4):241–6.

[68] Gwyn K. Children exposed to chemotherapy in utero. J Natl Cancer Inst Monogr 2005;(34): 69–71.

[69] Beral V, Bull D, Doll R, et al. Breast cancer and abortion: collaborative reanalysis of data from 53 epidemiological studies, including 83,000 women with breast cancer from 16 countries. Lancet 2004;363(9414):1007–16.

[70] Haagensen C. Carcinoma of the breast in pregnancy. In: Diseases of the breast. 2nd edition. Philadelphia: WB Saunders; 1971. p. 660–8.

[71] Peters M. The effect of pregnancy in breast cancer. In: Forrest A, Kunkler P, editors. Prognostic factors in breast cancer. Baltimore: Williams and Wilkins; 1968. p. 65–80.

[72] Greene F, Leis H. Management of breast cancer in pregnancy: a thirty-five year multi-institutional experience. Proc ASCO 1989;8:25.

[73] Ribeiro GG, Palmer MK. Breast carcinoma associated with pregnancy: a clinician's dilemma. BMJ 1977;2(6101):1524–7.

[74] Upponi SS, Ahmad F, Whitaker IS, et al. Pregnancy after breast cancer. Eur J Cancer 2003; 39(6):736–41.

ELSEVIER
SAUNDERS

Obstet Gynecol Clin N Am
32 (2005) 559–568

OBSTETRICS AND
GYNECOLOGY
CLINICS
OF NORTH AMERICA

# Malignant Melanoma in Pregnancy

Charles L. Wiggins, PhD[a,b,c,*],
Marianne Berwick, PhD, MPH[a,c],
Julia A. Newton Bishop, MD[d]

[a]Division of Epidemiology, Department of Internal Medicine, MSC-10 5550,
1 University of New Mexico, Albuquerque, NM 87131-0001, USA
[b]New Mexico Tumor Registry, MSC-11 6020, 1 University of New Mexico, Albuquerque,
NM 87131–0001, USA
[c]Epidemiology and Cancer Prevention, University of New Mexico Cancer Research and
Treatment Center, MSC 08 4630, 1 University of New Mexico, Albuquerque, NM 87131–0001, USA
[d]Genetic Epidemiology Division, Cancer Research, Cancer Genetics Building,
St. James's University Hospital, Beckett Street, Leeds LS9 7TF, UK

Malignant melanoma arises from melanocytes, cells of neural crest origin that produce the pigment melanin [1,2]. Incidence rates for malignant melanoma have increased dramatically in recent decades, both in the United States [3] and in other countries [4]. The American Cancer Society estimates that approximately 60,000 new cases of cutaneous malignant melanoma will be diagnosed in the United States during calendar year 2005 [5].

Incidence rates for malignant melanoma are highest among whites [3,4]. Exposure to solar ultraviolet radiation is considered to be the primary risk factor for the disease in fair-skinned populations [6,7]. Melanoma is relatively rare among Asians, blacks, American Indians, Hispanics, and other people of color [3,4,8]. Further, the histologic and primary site distribution of melanomas among whites differs from those of other populations [8–11].

Concern regarding the possible association between pregnancy and development of malignant melanoma arose from early case reports of aggressive disease

This work was supported by Contract No. N01-PC-35138 from the National Cancer Institute and by Institutional Research Grant IRG-92-024-10 from the American Cancer Society.

* Corresponding author. New Mexico Tumor Registry, MSC-11 6020, 1 University of New Mexico, Albuquerque, NM 87131–0001.

E-mail address: cwiggins@salud.unm.edu (C.L. Wiggins).

that was observed in pregnant women [12–14]. Such concern persists despite contrary evidence that emerged in intervening decades [15,16]. There are many excellent and detailed reviews of this topic in the medical literature [15–17]. This article provides a concise overview of issues relating to melanoma and pregnancy, including pregnancy-associated risk and prognosis, and briefly summarizes results from relevant reports that have been published in recent years.

## Background

Interest in the possible deleterious effects of pregnancy on occurrence and prognosis of melanoma primarily stemmed from the following observations: (1) case reports of aggressive disease in pregnant women; (2) melanoma incidence rates that are higher for females than males during the reproductive years; (3) cutaneous hyperpigmentation associated with both pregnancy and use of exogenous hormones; (4) reported differences in survival between pregnant and nonpregnant women with melanoma; and (5) results from studies that reported associations between use of exogenous hormones and occurrence of melanoma. These factors are introduced in the following paragraphs and are further discussed in subsequent sections of this manuscript.

### Case reports

Case reports of aggressive melanoma among pregnant women raised concern that factors associated with pregnancy increased the risk of developing or dying from the disease. For example, Pack and Scharnagel [12] published a report of 1050 individuals with malignant melanoma; 10 cases arose during pregnancy and half of these individuals died within 3 years of diagnosis. Such reports were subsequently criticized for having lacked appropriate control groups and for failing to adjust for prognostic determinants, such as tumor thickness and stage of disease at diagnosis.

### Incidence rates

Most cases of malignant melanoma in the general population occur among men and there is a corresponding male preponderance in the age-adjusted incidence rates of the disease [3]. With the exception of early childhood, however, age-specific incidence rates are higher among females than males during the first four decades of life (Fig. 1), roughly corresponding to a period when female reproductive hormones are most active. In several areas of Europe, such as the United Kingdom, the incidence of melanoma is higher in women at all ages. This observation is consistent with the hypothesis that hormones may play a role in the etiology of the disease [18].

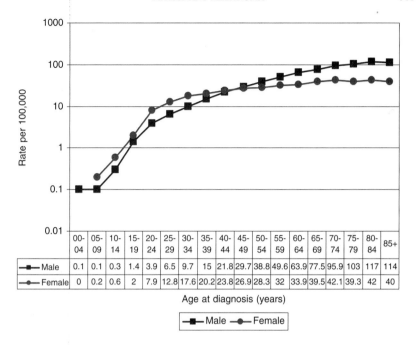

| | 00-04 | 05-09 | 10-14 | 15-19 | 20-24 | 25-29 | 30-34 | 35-39 | 40-44 | 45-49 | 50-54 | 55-59 | 60-64 | 65-69 | 70-74 | 75-79 | 80-84 | 85+ |
|---|---|---|---|---|---|---|---|---|---|---|---|---|---|---|---|---|---|---|
| ■ Male | 0.1 | 0.1 | 0.3 | 1.4 | 3.9 | 6.5 | 9.7 | 15 | 21.8 | 29.7 | 38.8 | 49.6 | 63.9 | 77.5 | 95.9 | 103 | 117 | 114 |
| ● Female | 0 | 0.2 | 0.6 | 2 | 7.9 | 12.8 | 17.6 | 20.2 | 23.8 | 26.9 | 28.3 | 32 | 33.9 | 39.5 | 42.1 | 39.3 | 42 | 40 |

Age at diagnosis (years)

■ Male ● Female

Fig. 1. Average annual age-specific incidence rates per 100,000 United States whites (SEER Program) diagnosed 1997 to 2001.

*Hyperpigmentation in pregnancy*

Many women experience a darkening of the skin on the face, abdomen, and other areas of the body during pregnancy, a condition known as "melasma" [19]. Melasma has also been associated with use of exogenous hormones [20,21]. Such evidence that melanocytes may be stimulated by hormones has fueled speculation that pregnancy-associated hormones could also influence the risk of melanoma.

*Differences in survival*

Early case reports suggested that women who were diagnosed with melanoma during or shortly after pregnancy had poor prognoses [12–14]. Again, interpretation of these reports is constrained because of lack of information regarding key prognostic factors and lack of appropriate control groups. Results from more recent studies that were based on relatively large numbers of cases, augmented with information on prognostic factors, suggest that pregnancy does not influence prognosis of melanoma.

*Reported associations between exogenous hormone use and melanoma*

Reports from three cohort studies conducted in the 1970s documented an increased risk for melanoma among women exposed to exogenous hormones

[22–24]. Most studies conducted since that time, however, reported equivocal findings: no association or risks that were restricted to defined subgroups [25,26].

## Pregnancy and risk of melanoma

Risk of developing malignant melanoma during pregnancy has been examined in relation to both maternal disease and deleterious effects on the infant. Previous studies of maternal risk of melanoma focused on the possible etiologic role of pregnancy-associated factors in development of the disease, and maternal prognosis. In contrast, studies of fetal risk of melanoma dealt with metastatic spread of maternal melanoma to the placenta and fetus, and subsequent prognosis of the offspring. These issues are addressed independently in the following sections.

### Risk of maternal melanoma during pregnancy

Malignant melanoma is often cited as one of the most common tumors reported in pregnancy [27,28]. It is important to recognize, however, that malignant melanoma is one of the most common types of cancer that occurs among white women during their childbearing years (Table 1). In the context of women in their childbearing years, the relevant research question is whether the risk of developing melanoma is greater for pregnant women than women who are not pregnant.

Reports from two population-based studies showed that the number of incident melanoma cases diagnosed among pregnant women did not exceed the number of such cases that would have been expected to occur based on prevailing incidence rates for the disease [29,30]; both studies were based on linkages between population registries of births and cancer. In a population-based study of Connecticut women who were diagnosed with melanoma while between the ages

Table 1
Most common primary cancer sites and types diagnosed among United States White women ages 15–44 years during the time period 1998–2002

| Age at diagnosis | Rank | Primary cancer site and type | Age-specific incidence rate[a] |
|---|---|---|---|
| 15–24 y | 1 | Thyroid | 6.5 |
| | 2 | Cutaneous melanoma | 5.4 |
| | 3 | Hodgkin lymphoma | 4.7 |
| 25–34 y | 1 | Breast | 16.9 |
| | 2 | Cutaneous melanoma | 15.8 |
| | 3 | Thyroid | 15.5 |
| 35–44 y | 1 | Breast | 92.7 |
| | 2 | Cutaneous melanoma | 22.6 |
| | 3 | Thyroid | 19.3 |

[a] Age-specific incidence rates per 100,000 for residents of nine core geographic areas that participate in the National Cancer Institute's Surveillance, Epidemiology, and End Results Program.

of 15 and 40 years, the observed number of pregnancies that occurred in the study group was approximately the same as would have been predicted based on corresponding birth rates; this observation was consistent with no excess of melanoma during pregnancy [31].

Several investigations were designed to examine possible associations between pregnancy-associated factors (eg, number of pregnancies, age at first pregnancy, number of live births, and number of miscarriages) and subsequent development of melanoma. Most studies found no evidence that factors linked to prior pregnancies increased subsequent risk of developing melanoma [32–38]. Associations between prior pregnancy and melanoma reported by some investigators were inconsistent across categories and were generally of modest magnitude [39,40].

Consistent evidence of an association between estrogens and melanoma has not emerged. Prentice and Thomas [25] systematically reviewed results from case-control and cohort studies that were conducted in the 1970s and 1980s to examine the association between use of oral contraceptives and melanoma. Results from most case-control studies showed no overall association between use of oral contraceptives and melanoma [32,33,35,41–44], although one study showed a modest positive association that did not achieve statistical significance [22]. Comparable evidence from three cohort studies reviewed by Prentice and Thomas [25] was inconsistent, with two studies showing modest positive associations between oral contraceptive use and melanoma (one statistically significant [24], the other not [23]) and the remaining study showing a nonsignificant protective effect of oral contraceptive use and melanoma [41]. There was some evidence that duration of oral contraceptive use was associated with melanoma [22,32,41,44], but such risk was not always dose dependent.

Karagas and colleagues [26] conducted a pooled-analysis of data from 10 case-control studies to examine the association between oral contraceptive use and melanoma. This analysis included 2391 cases and 3199 controls from various countries. The pooled odds ratio for the association between exogenous hormone use for 1 year or longer compared with never use or use less than 1 year was 0.86 (95% confidence interval 0.74–1.01); there was no evidence of heterogeneity between studies. These investigators found no relation between melanoma incidence and duration of oral contraceptive use, age began, year of use, years since first use or last use, or specifically current oral contraceptive use.

Duration of oral contraceptive use was related to melanoma in data from the Nurse's Health study [45]. Two other studies found no such association [39,46].

*Pregnancy and maternal prognosis from melanoma*

The possible influence of pregnancy on survival from melanoma is most appropriately considered in the context of well-established prognostic factors for the disease [47]. Melanoma prognosis is strongly associated with Breslow thickness, which is measured as the depth of the lesion from the granular cell layer of the epidermis to the deepest easily identifiable tumor cells [47,48]. Anatomic site of the melanoma has also been associated with prognosis; lesions occurring on the head, neck, and trunk generally have worse survival than those at other sites [49]. Presence of tumor ulceration is also associated with poor prognosis [49].

Some early reports of poor prognosis among pregnant women with melanoma were based on relatively small numbers of cases, did not control for recognized prognostic factors, and did not always identify an appropriate control group [12–14]. In contrast, five studies conducted in the 1970s, 1980s, and 1990s were well equipped to address the effects of pregnancy on melanoma prognosis [50–54]. These studies had well-defined case and control groups and ascertained relevant information about multiple prognostic factors for melanoma. In each of these studies, there was no significant difference in overall survival between melanoma cases diagnosed during pregnancy and their respective control groups. In four of these studies [50,52–54], women who developed melanoma during pregnancy had thicker tumors than the controls and were more likely to develop recurrent disease. Nonetheless, overall survival did not significantly vary among cases and controls in these studies.

Results summarized in three recent reports are compelling because each study was based on a relatively large number of cases and controls, and two of the three studies were population-based and may have been less affected by selection biases that may have accrued in clinic-based studies. Daryanani and colleagues [55] reported no difference in overall survival and disease-free survival between women who developed melanoma during pregnancy and an age-matched comparison group of women who were not pregnant when diagnosed with melanoma. The study was based on pregnant and nonpregnant women with melanoma who were seen at a large medical center in The Netherlands during the time period 1965 to 2001. The report was restricted to individuals with stage I and II melanoma; individuals with stage III and IV disease were excluded because the small number of such cases precluded meaningful statistical analyses. Pregnant (N = 46) and nonpregnant (N = 368) subjects with stage I and II melanoma did not differ by location of tumor, histologic type, tumor ulceration, or vascular invasion. Pregnancy was associated with a deeper Breslow thickness (2 mm in the pregnant group and 1.7 mm in the nonpregnant group), although this observation was not statistically significant.

Results from a retrospective cohort study of all Swedish women who were diagnosed with cutaneous melanoma during their reproductive years were recently reported by Lens and coworkers [56]. The study cohort included 185 women who were diagnosed with melanoma during pregnancy and 5348 women of comparable age who were not pregnant at the time of melanoma diagnosis. The investigators found no significant difference in overall survival between the pregnant and nonpregnant groups (log rank test, $P = .361$). Pregnancy was not a significant predictor of survival in a Cox proportional hazards model that simultaneously controlled for Breslow thickness, tumor site, Clark's level, and age (hazard ratio = 1.08, 95% confidence interval 0.60–1.93).

O'Meara and colleagues [57] linked records from independent, population-based records of cancer and births in California to characterize melanomas that occurred among women of childbearing age during the time period 1991 to 1999. In a Cox proportional hazards model that simultaneously controlled for age, race, stage, and tumor thickness, women who developed melanoma during or immediately following pregnancy had slightly better survival than nonpregnant women who developed the disease; this observation was not statistically significant. There was also no difference between pregnant and nonpregnant women with melanoma with regard to tumor thickness, stage of disease at diagnosis, anatomic site of tumor, or histology.

*Fetal and infant melanoma caused by metastasis*

There has been no population-based investigation of melanomas that arose from metastasis of maternal melanoma to the fetus. Rather, present knowledge of this subject is based solely on case reports and systematic reviews of case reports that have been published in the medical literature [58–61]. The relatively small number of case reports that have been reported in the medical literature suggest that congenital melanoma arising from maternal metastasis is an extremely rare phenomenon. Existing case reports also suggest that melanomas that are diagnosed in utero tend to have a poor prognosis.

## Summary

The bulk of evidence amassed over the past half century suggests that pregnancy does not significantly affect the risk of developing malignant melanoma. Further, pregnancy does not seem adversely to influence overall survival from the disease. Results from some studies suggested that pregnant women with melanoma were more likely than their nonpregnant counterparts to exhibit adverse prognostic indicators, such as thicker lesions and shorter time to recurrence. Nonetheless, most studies found no difference in overall survival between pregnant and nonpregnant women with melanoma. Recent reports from large-scale, population-based studies support these conclusions.

## References

[1] Urist MM, Heslin MJ, Miller DM. Malignant melanoma. In: Lenhard Jr RE, Osteen RT, Gansler T, editors. Clinical oncology. Malden (MA): American Cancer Society/Blackwell Science; 2001. p. 553–61.

[2] Morton DL, Essner R, Kirkwood JM, et al. Malignant melanoma. In: Bast Jr RC, Kufe DW, Pollock RE, et al, editors. Cancer medicine. 5th edition. Hamilton, Ontario, Canada: American Cancer Society/BC Decker; 2000. p. 1849–69.

[3] Ries LAG, Eisner MP, Kosary CL, et al, editors. SEER cancer statistics review, 1975–2002. National Cancer Institute, Bethesda, MD. Available at: http://seer.cancer.gov/csr/1975_2002/, based on November 2004 SEER data submission, posted to the SEER web site 2005. Accessed May 1, 2005.

[4]  Parkin DM, Whelan SL, Ferlay J, et al. Cancer incidence in five continents, vol. 8. IARC Scientific Publication No. 155. Lyon, France: International Agency for Research on Cancer; 2002.

[5]  American Cancer Society. Cancer facts and figures 2005. Atlanta, Georgia, 2005. Available at: http://www.cancer.org/. Accessed May 1, 2005.

[6]  English DR, Armstrong BK, Kricker A, et al. Sunlight and cancer. Cancer Causes Control 1997;8:271–83.

[7]  Armstrong BK, Kricker A. How much melanoma is caused by sun exposure? Melanoma Res 1993;3:395–401.

[8]  Cress RD, Holly EA. Incidence of cutaneous melanoma among non-Hispanic whites, Hispanics, Asians, and blacks: an analysis of California Cancer Registry data, 1983–93. Cancer Causes Control 1997;8:246–52.

[9]  Bergfelt L, Newell GL, Sider JG, et al. Incidence and anatomic distribution of cutaneous melanoma among United States Hispanics. J Surg Oncol 1989;40:222–6.

[10]  Black WC, Goldhahn RT, Wiggins CL. Melanoma within a Southwestern Hispanic population. Arch Dermatol 1987;123:1331–4.

[11]  Black WC, Wiggins C. Melanoma among Southwestern American Indians. Cancer 1985;55: 2899–902.

[12]  Pack GT, Scharnagel IM. Prognosis for malignant melanoma in the pregnant woman. Cancer 1951;4:324–34.

[13]  Byrd Jr FJ, McGanity WJ. Effect of pregnancy on the clinical course of malignant melanoma. South Med J 1954;47:196–200.

[14]  Riberti C, Marola G, Bertani A. Malignant melanoma: the adverse effect of pregnancy. Br J Plast Surg 1981;34:338–9.

[15]  Katz VL, Farmer RM, Dotters D. From nevus to neoplasm: myths of melanoma in pregnancy. Obstet Gynecol Surv 2002;57:112–9.

[16]  Grin CM, Driscoll MS, Grant-Kels JM. The relationship of pregnancy, hormones, and melanoma. Semin Cutan Med Surg 1998;17:167–71.

[17]  Driscoll MS, Grin-Jorgensen CM, Grant-Kels JM. Does pregnancy influence the prognosis of malignant melanoma? J Am Acad Dermatol 1993;29:619–30.

[18]  Sadoff L, Winkley J, Tyson S. Is malignant melanoma an endocrine dependent tumor? Oncology 1973;27:244–57.

[19]  Grimes PE. Melasma: etiologic and therapeutic considerations. Arch Dermatol 1995;131:1453–7.

[20]  Goh CL, Dlova CN. A retrospective study on the clinical presentation and treatment outcome of melasma in a tertiary dermatological referral centre in Singapore. Singapore Med J 1999;40: 455–8.

[21]  Resnick S. Melasma induced by oral contraceptive drugs. JAMA 1967;199:95–9.

[22]  Beral V, Ramcharan S, Faris R. Malignant melanoma and oral contraceptive use among women in California. Br J Cancer 1977;36:804–9.

[23]  Kay CR. Malignant melanoma and oral contraceptives. Br J Cancer 1981;44:479.

[24]  Ramcharan S, Pellegrin FA, Ray R, et al. The Walnut Creek Contraceptive Drug Study: a prospective study of the side effects of oral contraceptives III. Washington, DC: US Government Printing Office; 1981. NIH Publication No. 81–564.

[25]  Prentice RL, Thomas DB. On the epidemiology of oral contraceptives and disease. Adv Cancer Res 1987;49:285–401.

[26]  Karagas MR, Stukel TA, Dykes J, et al. A pooled analysis of 10 case-control studies of melanoma and oral contraceptive use. Br J Cancer 2002;86:1085–92.

[27]  Weisz B, Schiff E, Lishner M. Cancer in pregnancy: maternal and fetal implications. Hum Reprod Update 2001;7:384–93.

[28]  Potter JF, Schoeneman M. Metastasis of maternal cancer to the placenta and fetus. Cancer 1970;25:380–8.

[29]  Lambe M, Ekbom A. Cancers coinciding with child bearing: delayed diagnosis during pregnancy? BMJ 1995;311:1607–8.

[30]  Haas JF. Pregnancy in association with a newly diagnosed cancer: a population-based epidemiologic assessment. Int J Cancer 1984;34:229–35.

[31] Houghton AN, Flannery J, Viola MV. Malignant melanoma of the skin occurring during pregnancy. Cancer 1981;48:407–10.

[32] Holly EA, Weiss NS, Liff JM. Cutaneous melanoma in relation to exogenous hormones and reproductive factors. J Natl Cancer Inst 1983;70:827–31.

[33] Holman CDJ, Armstrong BK, Heenan PF. Cutaneous malignant melanoma in women: exogenous sex hormones and reproductive factors. Br J Cancer 1984;50:673–80.

[34] Green A, Bain C. Hormonal factors and melanoma in women. Med J Aust 1985;142:446–8.

[35] Gallagher RP, Elwood JM, Hill GB, et al. Reproductive factors, oral contraceptives and risk of malignant melanoma: Western Canada Melanoma Study. Br J Cancer 1985;52:901–7.

[36] Østerlind A, Tucker MA, Stone BJ, et al. The Danish case-control study of cutaneous malignant melanoma. III. Hormonal and reproductive factors in women. Int J Cancer 1988;42:821–4.

[37] Zanetti R, Franceschi S, Rosso S, et al. Cutaneous malignant melanoma in females: the role of hormonal and reproductive factors. Int J Epidemiol 1990;19:522–6.

[38] Holly EA, Cress RD, Ahn DK. Cutaneous melanoma in women. III. Reproductive factors and oral contraceptive use. Am J Epidemiol 1995;141:943–50.

[39] Smith MA, Fine JA, Barnhill RL, et al. Hormonal and reproductive influences and risk of melanoma in women. Int J Epidemiol 1998;27:751–7.

[40] Beral V. Parity and susceptibility to cancer. Ciba Found Symp 1983;96:182–203.

[41] Adam SA, Sheaves JK, Wright NH, et al. A case-control study of the possible association between oral contraceptives and malignant melanoma. Br J Cancer 1981;44:45–50.

[42] Bain C, Hennekens CH, Speizer FE, et al. Oral contraceptive use and malignant melanoma. J Natl Cancer Inst 1982;68:537–9.

[43] Helmrick SP, Rosenberg L, Kaufman DW, et al. Lack of an elevated risk of malignant melanoma in relation to oral contraceptive use. J Natl Cancer Inst 1984;72:617–20.

[44] Beral V, Evans S, Shaw H, et al. Oral contraceptive use and malignant melanoma in Australia. Br J Cancer 1984;50:681–5.

[45] Feskanich D, Hunter DJ, Willett WC, et al. Oral contraceptive use and risk of melanoma in premenopausal women. Br J Cancer 1999;81:918–23.

[46] Westerdahl J, Olsson H, Masback A, et al. Risk of malignant melanoma in relation to drug intake, alcohol, smoking and hormonal factors. Br J Cancer 1996;73:1126–31.

[47] Balch CM, Soong SJ, Gershenwald JE, et al. A prognostic factors analysis of 17,600 melanoma patients: validation of the American Joint Committee on Cancer melanoma staging system. J Clin Oncol 2001;19:3622–34.

[48] Breslow A. Thickness, cross-sectional areas and depth of invasion in the prognosis of cutaneous melanoma. Ann Surg 1970;172:902–8.

[49] Stadelmann WK, Rapaport DP, Soong S-J, et al. Prognostic, clinical, and pathologic features. In: Balch CM, Houghton AN, Sober AJ, et al, editors. Cutaneous melanoma. 3rd edition. St. Louis: Quality Medical Publishing; 1998. p. 11–35.

[50] Reintgen DS, McCarty KS, Vollmer R, et al. Malignant melanoma and pregnancy. Cancer 1985;55:1340–4.

[51] Wong JH, Sterns EE, Kopald KH, et al. Prognostic significance of pregnancy in stage I melanoma. Arch Surg 1989;124:1227–31.

[52] Slingluff CL, Reintgen DS, Vollmer RT, et al. Malignant melanoma arising during pregnancy: a study of 100 patients. Ann Surg 1990;211:552–9.

[53] MacKie RM, Bufalino R, Morabito A, et al. Lack of effect of pregnancy on outcome of melanoma. Lancet 1991;337:653–5.

[54] Travers RL, Sober AJ, Berwick M, et al. Increased thickness of pregnancy-associated melanoma. Br J Dermatol 1995;132:876–83.

[55] Daryanani D, Plukker JT, De Hullu JA, et al. Pregnancy and early-stage melanoma. Cancer 2003;97:2248–53.

[56] Lens MB, Rosdahl I, Ahlbom A, et al. Effect of pregnancy on survival in women with cutaneous malignant melanoma. J Clin Oncol 2004;22:4369–75.

[57] O'Meara AT, Cress R, Xing G, et al. Malignant melanoma in pregnancy: a population-based evaluation. Cancer 2005;103:1217–26.

[58] Richardson SK, Tannous ZS, Mihm Jr MC. Congenital and infantile melanoma: review of the literature and report of an uncommon variant, pigment-synthesizing melanoma. J Am Acad Dermatol 2002;47:77–90.

[59] Alexander A, Samlowski WE, Grossman D, et al. Metastatic melanoma in pregnancy: risk of transplacental metastases in the infant. J Clin Oncol 2003;21:2179–86.

[60] Baergen RN, Johnson D, Moore T, et al. Maternal melanoma metastatic to the placenta: a case report and review of the literature. Arch Pathol Lab Med 1997;121:508–11.

[61] Dildy III GA, Moise Jr KJ, Carpenter Jr RJ, et al. Maternal malignancy metastatic to the products of conception: a review. Obstet Gynecol Surv 1989;44:535–40.

ELSEVIER
SAUNDERS

Obstet Gynecol Clin N Am
32 (2005) 569–593

OBSTETRICS AND
GYNECOLOGY
CLINICS
OF NORTH AMERICA

# Malignant Adnexal Masses in Pregnancy

Hamid Sayar, MD[a], Catherine Lhomme, MD[b],
Claire F. Verschraegen, MD[a],*

[a]Cancer Research and Treatment Center, Division of Hematology Oncology,
University of New Mexico, 900 Camino de Salud, NE, Albuquerque, NM 87131, USA
[b]Institut Gustave Roussy, Villejuif, France

Ovarian tumors during pregnancy are very rare; however, a cancer diagnosis causes distress to the couple. Reassurance is paramount, and the first consideration should be given to the safety of the mother. If both mother and fetus can be preserved, treatment to minimize the risks to both should be planned accordingly. It is imperative to care for the patient with a multidisciplinary team that includes a high-risk obstetrician, a gynecologic oncologist, and a medical oncologist specialized in gynecologic cancers.

## Malignant adnexal masses in pregnancy

### Epidemiology

A review of 21 publications from 1954 to 1998 shows that the reported incidence of adnexal mass during pregnancy ranges from 1 in 79 to 1 in 2334, which averages at 1 in 800 [1–22]. This significant variation is the result of differences in the detection methods, the study population, and what types of masses are reported. In the same series of reports, malignant masses comprised from 0.8% to 10% of the adnexal masses, with an average of 5%. One can calculate from these numbers that, on average, 1 in 16,000 pregnancies is complicated with a malignant adnexal mass. The low incidence of ovarian neoplasia during preg-

---

* Corresponding author.
*E-mail address:* cverschraegen@salud.unm.edu (C.F. Verschraegen).

nancy reflects the low prevalence of invasive epithelial ovarian cancers at this young age.

## Clinical presentation

A significant number of pregnant women with an adnexal mass are asymptomatic. The mass is usually found on routine physical examination, during ultrasound, or at the time of caesarean section [23]. Those who are symptomatic mostly present with acute or chronic abdominal pain; others have obstetric complications, mainly obstructed labor, or other problems, such as increasing abdominal girth [24,25].

## Diagnosis and differential diagnosis

Imaging diagnosis of adnexal mass during pregnancy is traditionally by ultrasonography. Simple, unilateral ovarian masses smaller than 5 cm during first trimester of pregnancy are mostly functional luteal cysts and usually become undetectable by 14 weeks' gestation. Adnexal masses greater than 5 cm, bilateral masses, those growing or persisting into the second trimester, and masses that appear with papillary projections, solid compartments, multicystic, or septated on ultrasonography need further investigation. Bromley and Benacerraf assessed the accuracy of sonographic examination to characterize adnexal masses during pregnancy [21]. This study evaluated 125 pregnant women beyond 12 weeks of gestation with 131 adnexal masses measuring 4 cm or greater. An average of 80% of benign lesions diagnosed by sonographic examination correlated with final pathologic findings. Ultrasonography, however, was less accurate in characterizing malignant lesions, because 14 (10.7%) of the 131 lesions had sonographic characteristics suggestive of malignancy but only one of them (7%) had ovarian cancer. MRI compares with ultrasonography in characterizing the nature of adnexal masses in pregnancy [26,27] and is useful further to identify the lesions that could not be accurately diagnosed by ultrasonography. CT should not be used in pregnant women. Eventually, the final definite diagnosis is conventionally made by pathologic examination.

In all cases, consultation with a gynecologic oncologist and a medical oncologist specialized in gynecologic cancers is warranted. Surgery should be performed by the gynecologic oncologist and chemotherapy, if indicated, should be administered by the medical oncologist. The oncology team must work in close contact with an obstetrician specialized in high-risk pregnancies.

## Pathologic types

Pathologically, germ cell tumors comprise 45% of ovarian malignancies diagnosed during pregnancy, followed by epithelial tumors (37.5%); sex cord–stromal tumors (10%); and miscellaneous pathologies (7.5%) [28]. Each neoplastic type is discussed later.

## Ovarian germ cell cancer during pregnancy

Both benign and malignant ovarian germ cell tumors occur primarily in young women [29]. There are different histologic types of malignant germ cell tumors: dysgerminoma; endodermal sinus (yolk sac) tumor; immature malignant teratoma; choriocarcinoma; embryonal carcinoma; polyembryoma; and mixed germ cell tumors.

### Dysgerminomas

Dysgerminoma is the most common germ cell malignancy [30], and because germ cell tumors are found mainly in young women, it is not surprising for dysgerminomas to be the most frequent ovarian cancer in pregnancy. Dysgerminomas are usually unilateral and most frequently solid tumors [31]. In approximately 10% to 15%, however, the opposite ovary may be involved [32]. The staging work-up should involve an imaging study of the para-aortic lymph nodes and the lungs.

### Pathology

Dysgerminoma is the equivalent in women of seminoma. Macroscopically, dysgerminomas appear as a lobulated structure, firm in consistency, and cream colored or pale tan [30]. On histologic examination, the dysgerminoma cells are dispersed in sheets or cords separated by scant fibrous stroma [31]. Dysgerminomas often contain syncytiotrophoblastic giant cells that produce placental alkaline phosphatase and lactate dehydrogenase (LDH) [33,34]. These two markers can be used for monitoring purposes. Classical tumor markers, such as CA 125, are usually elevated during pregnancy and vary with the stage of pregnancy. Monitoring of the CA 125 is less useful during pregnancy.

### Presentation

Karlen and coworkers [35] in 1979 reviewed a total of 27 reported cases of dysgerminomas during pregnancy. All cases presented with a large-sized tumor ranging from 12 to 28 cm, and most of them were reportedly in early stage disease, 23 (85%) out of 27 being stage IA, although appropriate staging procedures to rule out distant small metastases had not been performed in many of these cases. Other case reports also indicate that dysgerminoma in pregnancy tends to be large, usually causing pain and abdominal distention more than expected for pregnancy age [36,37]. Because of the considerable size, these tumors are reported to be associated with obstetric complications, such as obstructed labor, cesarean section, or even fetal death.

### Treatment

The first step in the treatment of dysgerminoma is surgery. Pregnant patients are not exempt from this rule. The general consensus is to pursue surgical exploration of suspicious masses during pregnancy. If evidence is convincing to perform surgery and there is no acute complication that warrants emergent surgery, it is usually delayed until 16 to 18 weeks' gestation [2,32]. At this time the pregnancy is minimally dependent on corpus luteum hormone production and the risk of spontaneous abortion is negligible. The commonly recommended surgical approach is a midline incision and avoidance of any uterine manipulation. The midline incision enables adequate staging and necessary debulking. Peritoneal washing should be collected and a frozen section performed to guide further approaches. Because most patients present with early stage disease, unilateral salpingo-oophorectomy with preservation of the contralateral ovary and uterus is usually adequate. Surgical approach for more advanced stages is an area of controversy; however, generally the opposite ovary and uterus can be preserved if gross metastatic disease is not found in these locations. Adequate staging should be performed, which includes omental and peritoneal biopsies and sampling of suspicious pelvic and periaortic lymph nodes. Because dysgerminomas first metastasize into the ipsilateral lymph nodes, in case of early stage disease the staging lymphadenectomy may be limited to para-aortic ipsilateral lymph nodes. Although there is a 10% to 15% incidence of bilateral ovarian dysgerminomas, the biopsy of the contralateral ovary is warranted only if the ovary seems to be affected by the disease [38].

Following initial surgical intervention and staging work-up, the question of adjuvant chemotherapy arises. Given the low recurrence rate of stage IA disease after surgical resection, and also the high (>75%) cure rate of recurrent dysgerminomas with radiation therapy and chemotherapy, further therapy may be safely skipped in pregnant patients [32]. Some authorities also consider the same approach for stage IB disease (bilateral ovarian involvement) [23].

Unfortunately, there is a lack of data in the literature with regards to adjuvant chemotherapy in advanced-stage dysgerminoma, probably because most cases present with early stage disease, and are managed only by surgical approach. Optimal medical treatment has not been defined for dysgerminoma, and often reports of chemotherapy in other types of germ cell tumors during pregnancy are extrapolated to dysgerminomas. The treatment of dysgerminoma should follow the treatment of seminoma in men, however, for which there is more published data given the higher incidence of this testicular cancer. Buller and coworkers [38] reported a patient with a case of stage IV dysgerminoma who was treated with combination of cisplatin and etoposide at 26 weeks' gestation and delivered a healthy infant at 38 weeks. Etoposide may not be the best drug to use in a highly curable cancer, because of its leukemogenic potential.

*Special considerations*

Follow-up of treated ovarian dysgerminomas during pregnancy is the same as in nonpregnant state, usually with periodic clinical examinations and appropriate imaging studies. Serum LDH levels are usually normal in pregnancy unless it is complicated by preeclampsia [39]. Some case reports have shown that LDH is elevated in patients with dysgerminoma [40–43]. Moreover, LDH isoenzyme fractions 1, 2, and 3 were high in some of these patients. Schwartz and Morris [33] reported four cases of dysgerminoma in whom serum LDH levels correlated with tumor size and stage of disease. Serum LDH can be used as an easily measurable marker to monitor response to treatment or recurrence of disease during and after pregnancy. There is no evidence of increased risk of recurrence with future pregnancies in these patients. Further pregnancies are not generally contraindicated.

*Endodermal sinus tumors*

Endodermal sinus tumors (yolk sac) comprise about one fifth of the ovarian germ cell tumors and are the second most common malignant tumor of the germ cell origin [31,44].

*Pathology*

Histologically, there are tubules or spaces lined by single layers of flattened cuboidal cells, reticular stroma, and scattered globules. Characteristically, there is a glomerulus-like structure composed of a central blood vessel covered by germ cells within a space lined by germ cells (Schiller-Duval body). In most cases this tumor produces alpha fetoprotein (APF), which could be used for monitoring purposes [45].

*Presentation*

There are less than 20 reports of endodermal sinus tumors associated with pregnancy in the literature [46–59]. A review by Elit and coworkers [54] in 1999 concluded that about 70% of patients present with the disease confined to the ovary (stage I), and they mostly have markedly elevated maternal serum AFP at presentation. AFP is usually elevated during pregnancy and the level varies with the stage of pregnancy. When AFP is produced by a tumor, however, expected AFP levels are higher than the levels observed during pregnancy. Follow-up of AFP for persistent or recurrent disease may pose a problem in pregnant women. These tumors grow rapidly; some cases develop serious symptoms within 24 hours to 1 week. As a result of this rapid growth, they may present with acute abdomen, torsion, or bleeding into the tumor [48,60,61]. Arima and coworkers [56] reported a pregnant woman with endodermal sinus tumor, presenting with virilization and elevated serum testosterone level. The histologic examination revealed accumulations of Leydig cells throughout the tumor.

*Treatment*

To ensure long-term survival and cure, the medical treatment of endodermal sinus tumors needs to be aggressive despite the pregnancy. Treatment with surgery alone yields a poor prognosis with 5-year survival rate of only 13% [61]. Fortunately this tumor is very sensitive to chemotherapy and combination chemotherapy can offer up to 80% long-term survival in early stage disease [62–65]. The best approach is early surgical resection followed by appropriate multiagent adjuvant chemotherapy. The surgical resection could be similar to dysgerminoma cases, including unilateral salpingo-oophorectomy, preservation of the uterus, and appropriate intraoperative staging. There are several reports of pregnant women with endodermal sinus tumor treated with combination chemotherapy who delivered normal infants [45,50–52,55,59]. The most used chemotherapy regimen has been the combination of bleomycin, etoposide, and cisplatin (BEP). There are, however, exceptions to this. Elit and coworkers [54] reported a pregnant woman who was treated with postoperative chemotherapy with BEP at 25 weeks' gestation and delivered an infant with ventriculomegaly and cerebral atrophy. Shimizu and coworkers [58] reported a patient with stage Ic endodermal sinus tumor who underwent surgical resection at 19 weeks of gestation but did not receive postoperative chemotherapy. She delivered a normal infant at 36 weeks by cesarean section. A second look at the time of delivery showed no signs of recurrence, and she received chemotherapy after delivery with no evidence of recurrence at 27 months after initial treatment. The decision to administer chemotherapy is based on tumor markers, with elevations of AFP and LDH being the witness of persistent disease.

*Special considerations*

Patients with ovarian endodermal sinus tumor diagnosed during pregnancy are followed similar to nonpregnant women. Serum AFP is elevated in most cases, and this marker may be used for monitoring purposes with the caveat that AFP levels vary physiologically during pregnancy.

Despite one report of a patient who during the first pregnancy was treated for endodermal sinus tumor, which recurred during the second pregnancy [46], there is no proven contraindication for future pregnancies in these patients. Physicians should advise patients not to start a new pregnancy within 2 years of completing the treatment for endodermal sinus tumor.

*Other malignant germ cell tumors*

Embryonal carcinoma comprises only 4% of all malignant ovarian germ cell tumors [66], followed by other types being very rare. The occurrence of these germ cell tumors during pregnancy is extremely rare, and not many cases have been reported in the literature [60,66–71]. These malignancies may occur as pure one germ cell–type or a combination of two or more of the germ cell elements, which is referred to as "mixed germ cell tumor."

*Presentation*

Similar to other ovarian malignancies, these tumors may present with abdominal symptoms or be found incidentally on physical examination and imaging studies. There are reports of elevation of tumor markers in some of these tumors. For example, maternal serum AFP may be significantly elevated in immature teratoma [70,71,73] and embryonal carcinoma [41].

## Treatment

Treatment consists of surgery followed by chemotherapy. Surgery is similar to dysgerminomas, which consists of unilateral salpingo-oophorectomy and intra-operative staging [72,73]. In nonpregnant women, BEP is the treatment of choice. Less frequently the combinations of vinblastine, bleomycin, and cisplatin or vin-cristine, dactinomycin, and cyclophosphamide are used for embryonal carcinoma, immature teratoma, and mixed germ cell tumors [32]. There are few case reports of chemotherapy for these tumor types in pregnancy. For example, Horbelt and coworkers [68] treated a mixed germ cell tumor during pregnancy with BEP and the woman delivered a normal infant at 39 weeks' gestation. BEP and the combi-nation of vinblastine, bleomycin, and cisplatin have been used in pregnancy to treat immature teratoma followed by delivery of normal babies [59,69].

## Special considerations

If maternal serum AFP is elevated at diagnosis, it may be used as a marker for follow-up with the same previously noted caveat. Human chorionic gonadotropin is not reliable. There is no information as to whether it is safe for these patients to become pregnant again, but there is no report of recurrent disease in future pregnancies in the literature.

## Borderline and invasive ovarian epithelial tumors during pregnancy

Very few pregnant women develop ovarian epithelial tumors because this is a disease of older women. Ovarian epithelial tumors can be benign, borderline (or of low malignant potential) which is a disease of younger women, or invasive, the most common tumor seen in older women. The different pathologic types of invasive ovarian cancer are serous (75%); mucinous (10%); endometrioid (10%); clear cell; transitional cell carcinoma; Brenner tumor; epidermal-stromal; undif-ferentiated; carcinosarcoma; and mesodermal mixed tumors. Borderline ovarian tumors are usually of the serous or mucinous types. The latter is further dis-tinguished in intestinal or endocervical subtypes.

## Invasive epithelial tumors

### Pathology

*Invasive serous tumors.*   These are the most common invasive epithelial ovarian neoplasms. Grossly, they appear as cystic structures. Histologically, the lining epithelium exhibits complex growth pattern, which is papillary in nature, with infiltration or frank effacement of the underlying stroma by solid tumor. The individual tumor cells display usual features of malignancy [31].

*Invasive mucinous tumors.*   Grossly, these tumors consist of multiple cysts with variable size. They tend to produce large cystic masses and usually have more cysts compared with the serous tumors. Histologically, these tumors contain solid compartments with conspicuous epithelial cell atypia and stratification, loss of glandular architecture, and necrosis. Pseudomyxoma peritonei, a condition some-times associated with mucinous ovarian tumors, consists of extensive mucinous ascites, cystic epithelial implants on the peritoneal surfaces, and adhesions [31]. Most commonly, this condition arises from the appendix, which must be examined concurrently.

*Invasive endometrioid tumors.*    Containing both solid and cystic areas, these tumors are grossly similar to serous and mucinous tumors. On histologic examination, these tumors exhibit glandular patterns with strong resemblance to endometrial carcinoma. Interestingly, approximately 15% of endometrioid carcinomas are accompanied by a carcinoma of the endometrium [31,74].

*Clear cell adenocarcinoma.*    These tumors can be predominantly cystic or solid. Histologically, the cells have abundant clear cytoplasm. In cystic type, the cells line the cystic spaces, whereas in the solid variety they are arranged in tubules or sheets [31].

*Transitional cell carcinoma.*    Their gross appearance is typically solid and cystic. Microscopically, they contain blunt, thick, and long papillary folds with fibro-vascular cores, lined by transitional-type epithelium resembling those lining the urinary bladder. Transitional cell carcinomas are frequently seen in association with other types of carcinoma, most often serous tumors [75].

*Malignant Brenner tumors.*    These are transitional cell carcinomas in which a benign or atypical proliferative adenofibromatous (Brenner) component is identified. The epithelial component of these tumors consists of nests of transitional cells [31,75].

*Presentation*

Epithelial tumors in nonpregnant patients usually present with abdominal distention, intra-abdominal pressure, vague pain, dyspepsia, urinary frequency, and other abdominal symptoms. The presentation in pregnant patients is similar to nonpregnant women, however, because all these symptoms may also occur in normal pregnancy. A high clinical suspicion with appropriate physical examination and complementary imaging studies are usually needed to make the diagnosis. About 65% of invasive serous tumors, 40% of endometrioid types, 16% of Brenner tumors, and 5% of invasive mucinous neoplasms are bilateral [31,75]. Unfortunately, because of their site and lack of symptoms in early stages, these tumors are usually diagnosed at advanced stage disease. CA 125 in pregnant women with malignant epithelial ovarian tumors may be elevated as observed in nonpregnant patients.

*Treatment*

In nonpregnant patients, the standard treatment for invasive epithelial ovarian cancer is initial debulking surgery followed by adjuvant chemotherapy. Surgery typically consists of laparotomy with total abdominal hysterectomy, bilateral salpingo-oophorectomy, and meticulous staging omentectomy and lymphadenectomy. This type of surgical approach during pregnancy is not possible unless the patient opts to terminate the pregnancy.

There are nine reports of chemotherapy for invasive epithelial ovarian tumors during pregnancy in the literature [76–84]. Five of these cases presented with stage III disease [76,77,81,83,84], whereas the staging is not reported for the other four patients. One patient was diagnosed in the first trimester [83], five in second trimester [76–78,80,82], and three in the third trimester of pregnancy [79,81,84]. In seven of these patients, unilateral salpingo-oophorectomy was performed as an initial surgery during pregnancy, and total abdominal hysterectomy with contralateral salpingo-oophorectomy was postponed until after delivery [77–81,83,84]. In the two other cases, the initial surgery during pregnancy consisted of ovarian cystectomy only, with the complete surgery performed after delivery [76,82]. All authors used platinum-based chemotherapy during pregnancy after the initial surgical intervention. Four of these patients were treated with two to seven cycles of combination of cisplatin and cyclophosphamide [76,77,79,80], one patient with two cycles of cisplatin and paclitaxel [81], one with six cycles of carboplatin and paclitaxel [83], one with three cycles of carboplatin and cyclophosphamide [79], one with four cycles of single-agent cisplatin [82], and one with two cycles of single-agent carboplatin [84]. Eight patients received different numbers of cycles of chemotherapy following the postdelivery surgery and one did not because she had received seven cycles of cisplatin and cyclophosphamide during pregnancy [76]. In most cases delivery was done by cesarean section. All infants were born with reasonable maturity, in a good condition, and without gross congenital anomalies. With the exception of one infant for whom a follow-up is not reported [80], others did well after several months of observation. One patient died of recurrent disease 29 months after delivery [81], but others were disease free with follow-up periods ranging from 12 to 36 months.

It may be cautiously concluded from the experience with this very limited number of reported cases that partial surgery with adjuvant platinum-based chemotherapy during pregnancy, followed by completion of the necessary surgical intervention and more cycles of chemotherapy after delivery to complete therapy, yields a reasonable prognosis with none or minimal adverse consequences for the infant. Because of the results of ICON 3, demonstrating equivalence between single-agent carboplatin and carboplatin combinations, it may be prudent to limit the chemotherapy to single-agent carboplatin during pregnancy, and consider adding paclitaxel after delivery. If the cancer is diagnosed during the early period of the first trimester, an initial complete staging and debulking surgery without preservation of the pregnancy followed by conventional chemotherapy is the most reasonable approach. In any case, the overall survival of patients with ovarian cancer is 30% to 25% at 5 years. There is no indication that it is different if the cancer arises during pregnancy [84].

*Special considerations*

In patients with stage 1A disease, unilateral resection with close observation may be considered. This strategy is similar in both pregnant and nonpregnant patients. It may be worthwhile to remove the primary tumor but to delay the full staging work-up until after delivery, or until the time of the cesarean section, especially if the tumor is diagnosed in the second half of the pregnancy. No chemotherapy is needed if the staging is not upgraded at pathologic examination.

During normal pregnancy, there is a slight increase of CA 125 up to the tenth week of gestation [85]. In cases of imminent abortion with vaginal spotting or bleeding between 4 and 12 weeks' gestation, the serum CA 125 is usually high [86,87]. Although useful in confirmed disease, an elevated CA 125 level during first trimester of pregnancy should be interpreted with caution.

*Borderline epithelial tumors*

*Pathology*

Grossly, these tumors may not be easily differentiated from their benign or invasive counterparts. Histologically, in contrast to the benign tumors they demonstrate papillary epithelial proliferation and atypia, but are distinguished from invasive types by their lack of stromal invasion [88,89]. The basal membrane is intact. Peritoneal implants are sometimes seen with borderline tumors, which in 20% of cases may show some degrees of stromal invasion [90]. Serous tumors comprise most borderline epithelial neoplasms. Mucinous type is second in frequency and can be of intestinal or endocervical subtype.

*Presentation*

Newly diagnosed borderline tumors are confined to the ovary in 70% to 75% of cases. Similar to other ovarian tumors, patients are most commonly asymptomatic and the adnexal mass is found during a regular pelvic examination or by routine imaging studies. Some patients, however, may have pain or other pelvic symptoms. Approximately 40% of serous borderline tumors and 6% of mucinous types are bilateral at presentation [75]. A retrospective study of 1069 epithelial borderline ovarian tumors in Japan showed that only about half of these patients presented with elevated CA 125 levels, and less than half of this group had levels higher than 100 U/mL [91].

*Treatment*

Similar to all other ovarian malignancies, the treatment of borderline epithelial tumors is primarily surgical. In the nonpregnant setting, a radical surgery including total abdominal hysterectomy, bilateral salpingo-oophorectomy, omentectomy, and appropriate staging is usually the standard surgical approach, although in very young women fertility considerations may limit the surgery depending on the actual findings. Surgical resection without adjuvant chemotherapy is usually sufficient in patients with noninvasive peritoneal implants, and the prognosis for this group of patients is generally favorable [89,92–95]. Adjuvant chemotherapy is usually recommended for tumors with invasive peritoneal implants because they carry a 30% risk of evolution into a more aggressive disease [89,93,96]. Patients with rapidly growing tumors or those who develop ascites may require adjuvant chemotherapy, although no randomized study has established a true benefit [32]. In the case of young patients, conservative surgery to preserve fertility [89,97–99] includes unilateral salpingo-oophorectomy, simple ovariectomy, or cystectomy with preservation of the uterus. This approach is acceptable mainly in cases of unilateral tumors but could also be used in cases of bilateral disease [100]. The conservative treatment leaves the patient with a 30% risk of recurrence, but the recurrences can be treated surgically and the overall survival is not adversely affected [101–103].

There are, unfortunately, not enough data regarding therapeutic approaches to borderline tumors during pregnancy [104–107]. Wang and coworkers [108] reported a pregnant woman with stage Ia mucinous borderline tumor diagnosed at 18 weeks of gestation. The patient was treated by unilateral salpingo-oophorectomy during pregnancy, no adjuvant chemotherapy was administered, and the patient delivered a normal term infant. Studzinski and coworkers [109] performed cystectomy at 16 weeks' gestation on a patient with stage Ia borderline epithelial tumor, no chemotherapy was given, and the patient delivered a normal term infant. The patient was followed after pregnancy and did not show recurrence up to the time of publication of the report. Mikami and coworkers [110] reported a patient with stage Ic serous borderline tumor who was treated at week 14 of gestation by unilateral salpingo-oophorectomy, wedge resection of the opposite ovary, and partial omentectomy. The patient delivered a normal term infant.

It can be concluded that borderline epithelial tumors of ovary at least in the case of early stage disease may be safely treated by conservative surgery during pregnancy. In the case of advanced disease and considering the indolent course of these malignancies, debulking surgery can probably be postponed until after delivery. The therapeutic decision, however, should be highly individualized. As far as chemotherapy is concerned, it is very rarely recommended, and if administered, the regimen is usually platinum-based combination chemotherapy [111–113].

*Special considerations*

Epithelial ovarian tumors of low malignant potential are indolent in nature. The prognosis for these tumors is very good even for advanced stages [32]. Recurrent cases first should be treated with repeated surgery.

CA 125 may or may not be elevated in borderline epithelial tumors. Compared with their invasive counterparts, a greater tumor burden is required to yield an elevated serum CA 125 level in borderline tumors. The CA 125 level does not correlate with the clinical stage. The marker is usually within normal range even in cases of relapse [114].

Conservative surgical approach for treatment of borderline epithelial tumors in young women results in acceptable fertility outcomes [102,115–118]. About one to two thirds of such women are able successfully to conceive [107,118].

## Sex cord–stromal tumors during pregnancy

Ovarian stroma is the source of these tumors, which primarily contain cells derived from the sex cord of the embryonic gonad or ordinary stromal cells. They are rarely found in pregnancy. These cell types mainly include granulosa cells; theca cells (luteinized cells in the stroma); Sertoli cells; Leydig cells; and fibroblasts. These tumors are composed of one or more cell types, and so are named based on their composing elements: (1) fibromas; (2) thecomas; (3) granulosa (or granulose-theca) cell tumors, a combination of granulosa and theca cells; (4) Sertoli-Leydig cell tumors, a combination of Sertoli and Leydig cells; and (5) gynandroblastoma, which is composed of granulosa and Sertoli-Leydig cell types. Fibromas and thecomas are always benign, and are not part of this discussion. The granulosa tumors are considered malignant, usually with a favorable prognosis. The Sertoli-Leydig types are usually considered low-grade malignant, although some can be extremely malignant, especially if they contain neuroblastic elements. Gynandroblastoma is generally a benign tumor, but can be expected to behave as a low-grade malignancy [32]. Among these three potentially malignant types, granulosa tumors are the most frequent type (70%); followed by Sertoli-Leydig tumors; and finally gynandroblastoma, which is very rare.

### Pathology

#### Granulosa cell tumors
Their gross appearance varies from solid to cystic structures with different sizes. Histologically, the granulosa cell component may present as small, cuboidal to polygonal cells, which spread in shape of cords, strands, or sheets. The theca (luteinized) cell component is in the form of sheets or clusters of cuboidal to polygonal cells [31,119]. The theca cells produce estrogen, so if they are present in significant quantity the patient may manifest estrogen-related clinical findings, which in pregnant women may not be distinguishable from physiologic changes of pregnancy. The granulosa cells produce inhibin and sometimes estrogens [120].

#### Sertoli-Leydig cell tumors
These tumors are grossly solid, usually lobulated with a smooth external surface. On microscopic examination, the well-differentiated tumors appear in the form of hollow or solid tubules composed of Sertoli or Leydig cells interspersed with a fibrous stroma, whereas the less differentiated histologic subtypes exhibit a

less structured appearance [31,119]. The Leydig cells if present may produce androgens, which can cause relevant clinical manifestations.

## Gynandroblastoma

These rare tumors consist of a mixture of Sertoli or Leydig cells and granulosa cells. They may produce androgens or estrogens and patients can present with hyperandrogen or hyperestrogen symptoms [121,122].

## Presentation

These tumors usually present with abdominal pain, torsion, and increase in abdominal girth. They are also associated with infertility. Similar to other ovarian tumors, they may be suspected by physical examination and imaging studies, but the final definite diagnosis always relies on histologic examination.

Patients with granulosa tumors may have hypersecretion of estrogens, which in nonpregnant women can cause menstrual irregularity, abnormal vaginal bleeding, and breast tenderness. In pregnant women these symptoms are usually masked by the normal hyperestrogen state of pregnancy. Sertoli-Leydig cell tumors often produce androgens, which may result in hirsutism or virilization in pregnant women [123,124]. The granulosa tumors are bilateral in 2% to 8% of cases, and Sertoli-Leydig cell tumors in less than 5% of patients [31,125–129]. Granulosa cell tumors present with stage I disease in 78% to 91% of cases [130]. Zaloudek and Norris [131] reported 64 intermediate and poorly differentiated neoplasms of Sertoli-Leydig cell tumors; 62 of them (97%) presented with stage I disease.

Young and coworkers [132] in 1984 reported a series of 36 pregnant patients with sex cord–stromal tumors. In this report, granulosa cell type was diagnosed in 17 patients, Sertoli-Leydig cell in 13, and 6 were of unclassified histology. Eleven patients presented with abdominal pain or swelling, five in shock, two patients with virilization symptoms, and one complained of vaginal bleeding. Four patients were asymptomatic, three of them had palpable mass on physical examination, and the mass in the other one was detected by ultrasound. In 13 patients the tumor was discovered at the time of cesarean section; five had dystocia and the tumors were found incidentally in the other eight patients. The tumors were at stage I in all these patients but 13 of the tumors had ruptured. Hematoperitoneum was present in seven cases. The tumor was unilateral in all but one patient.

There is only one report of gynandroblastoma associated with pregnancy in the literature. This patient presented with a progressively enlarging, unilocular left ovarian cyst [133].

## Treatment

Most patients with sex cord–stromal tumors present with stage I disease, and generally these neoplasms have a low-grade malignancy nature. Conservative surgical intervention, including unilateral salpingo-oophorectomy, is the recommended initial approach to treat young patients with stage I disease [32,130]. Conservative surgical intervention in pregnant patients helps secure the pregnancy and fetus and future fertility. In case of more advanced disease, adjuvant chemotherapy should be considered [32,130,132,134]. Currently, in the non-pregnant patients, the recommended chemotherapy regimen for granulosa cell tumors is BEP [130,135–138]. BEP has been used in other ovarian malignancies during pregnancy with no major adverse effects on the second- and third-trimester fetus. This regimen may be considered in pregnancy settings if deemed necessary. For Sertoli-Leydig cell tumors in the nonpregnant setting, usually BEP or rarely vincristine, dactinomycin, and cyclophosphamide is being used [32,136]. BEP regimen may be considered in pregnant women with advanced Sertoli-Leydig cell tumors. One should always remember the risk of leukemia associated with etoposide.

For the only reported case of gynandroblastoma in pregnancy, unilateral salpingo-oophorectomy was performed after delivery, and a laparoscopic examination 1 year after surgery did not show any evidence of recurrent disease [133].

*Special considerations*

There are six nonneoplastic ovarian lesions associated with pregnancy that can simulate a malignancy on clinical and pathologic examination [139]. These lesions must be carefully evaluated and ruled out when malignant neoplasm is suspected. They include pregnancy luteoma, hyperreactio luteinalis, large solitary luteinized follicle cyst of pregnancy and puerperium, intrafollicular granulosa cell proliferations, hilus cell hyperplasia, and ectopic decidua. These lesions usually disappear spontaneously after termination of pregnancy or could be adequately treated by local surgical resection.

Inhibin, a polypeptide normally produced by the granulosa cells of ovarian follicles, has been shown to be elevated in granulosa cell tumors [140,141]. Elevated inhibin levels may also be observed in mucinous epithelial ovarian malignancies, so it is not specific [142]. There is an alpha type, available for detection in most laboratories, and a beta type probably more specific but still experimental.

Mullerian inhibitory substance, which is also referred to as "antimüllerian hormone," has been studied as a sensitive and specific tumor marker for granulosa cell tumors, and shown to be useful to evaluate the efficacy of treatment and to detect early recurrences [143,144]. This test is not routinely used.

## Carcinosarcoma of the ovary during pregnancy

Carcinosarcoma of the ovary, also known as "malignant mixed mesodermal tumor," is a rare clinical entity that is seen mainly in postmenopausal women. The prognosis is generally poor even with aggressive treatment [145–147]. There are only three cases of malignant mixed mesodermal tumor during pregnancy reported in the literature [148–150].

## Pathology

These tumors contain both malignant epithelial and mesenchymal (sarcoma) components [151]. These tumors sometimes contain malignant stromal structures, which are not normally found in the ovary [152]. Some reported examples of these abnormal sarcomatous elements are chondrosarcoma, rhabdomyosarcoma, leiomyosarcoma, and endometrioid stromal sarcoma [153].

## Presentation

In nonpregnant women, the most common clinical presentation is abdominal distention with or without a palpable pelvic or abdominal mass. Widespread metastases at the time of diagnosis or surgery are more common than other types of ovarian cancer [154,155].

## Treatment

There is no role for conservative surgical approach against this malignancy. An optimal debulking at the time of initial surgery is an extremely important determinant of the prognosis [155]. Aggressive chemotherapy following the initial surgery is essential. Several different combination chemotherapies have been attempted with low overall success rate. Le and coworkers [156] retrospectively reviewed the results of treatment with a combination of cisplatin and doxorubicin in 29 patients. This regimen, when given after initial aggressive surgical resection, was able to confer a median survival of 3 years, which was significantly superior to the previous treatments. There are also reports of a limited number of patients who demonstrated good response to a combination of doxorubicin, ifosfamide, and dacarbazine [157,158].

## Metastatic tumors to the ovary during pregnancy

Metastatic malignancies to the ovaries are not uncommon. They may be symptomatic, or found on pelvic examination or at the time of surgery; some of them may be microscopic and discovered only at the time of autopsy. Both gynecologic and nongynecologic malignancies can metastasize to the ovaries. In a study of 64 patients in Japan, 60% of metastatic ovarian tumors were from nongynecologic sources and 40% were gynecologic in origin [159]. In the United States these tumors are most commonly metastasized from colon or breast malignancies, whereas gastric cancer is the most frequent primary site in Japan, because of the high incidence of gastric cancer in that country [32,159]. Other reported primary sites of nongynecologic malignancies with metastases to ovaries include both adenocarcinoma and carcinoid of the appendix, small bowel, gallbladder, biliary duct, urinary bladder, ureter, and lung [159–166]. Carcinoid tumors and non-Hodgkin's lymphomas primarily arising in ovaries have also been reported by many different authors [167–171]. Struma ovarii is a neoplasm containing thyroid tissue, which could cause hyperthyroidism. There are reports of various primary cancers metastatic to the ovary in pregnancy [172–186].

*Pathology*

Generally, the histology of metastatic tumor is similar to the primary malignancy. In some cases, however, it may not be easy to distinguish between primary ovarian tumors and metastatic ones. In particular, diagnosis of metastatic colon malignancies to the ovaries may be difficult. It has been reported that up to 45% of metastatic colon tumors to the ovaries may be misdiagnosed as primary ovarian cancers [187,188]. The use of special cytokeratin stains helps the differential diagnosis.

Krukenberg tumors are common among metastatic tumors to the ovaries. They are adenocarcinomas with distinctive histologic features. These tumors originate usually from a gastric adenocarcinoma or an appendiceal carcinoma, but may occasionally originate from other sites, including colon, gallbladder, urinary bladder, cervix, and breast [166]. In some cases the primary site is unknown, a condition called "primary Krukenberg tumor." Yakushiji and coworkers [180] in a review of 112 Krukenberg tumors did not find the original site in about 30% of cases. Grossly, Krukenberg tumors are in the form of solid tumors. On histologic examination typical malignant cells often have a signet-ring appearance with vacuolated cytoplasm. These epithelial cells may demonstrate glandular or tubular appearance. The stroma has variable cellularity with spindle-shaped stromal cells [166]. The prognosis is very poor.

*Presentation*

The clinical presentation of metastatic tumors is similar to other ovarian neoplasms. Patients may present with acute or chronic abdominal symptoms, or the tumor can be found incidentally on physical examination, staging imaging studies, or even at the time of surgery. Interestingly, when occurring during pregnancy, some of these tumors manifest with masculinization or virilization of the mother or the fetus [189–195]. In a study of 12 cases of metastatic tumors to ovaries, 9 (75%) of them were bilateral [163]. At least 80% of Krukenberg tumors are bilateral [196].

*Treatment*

There is no single modality for the treatment of these tumors. Each patient is usually treated based on the type of the primary malignancy, also some of these tumors are diagnosed after surgical resection of the ovaries. For the same reason, the treatment of such tumors during pregnancy is usually individualized based on different factors including histologic type, gestational week, and patient's wishes.

## Clinical recommendations

Ovarian tumors during pregnancy are very rare. A cancer diagnosis, however, causes a lot of distress to the couple. Reassurance is paramount, and the first consideration should be given to the safety of the mother. If both mother and fetus can be preserved, treatment to minimize the risks to both should be planned accordingly. It is imperative to care for the patient with a multidisciplinary team that includes a high-risk obstetrician, a gynecologic oncologist, and a medical oncologist specialized in gynecologic cancers.

The most common tumors are germ cell tumors and borderline epithelial tumors. The standard treatment approach followed for a nonpregnant patient should be used in pregnancy. For germ cell tumors, surgery should be performed first. Not all germ cell tumors require chemotherapy. If the tumor occurs during the first trimester, consideration of chemotherapy should be delayed at least until the second trimester. In the case of rapidly growing tumors, a therapeutic abortion should be offered to the patient. The number of cycles of BEP should be planned with the term of the pregnancy. The pregnancy must be monitored very closely to prevent placental atrophy or fetal growth delay.

Borderline tumors are usually treated by surgery only, and because they are slow growing, consideration may be given to delaying treatment until delivery. Common invasive epithelial ovarian cancer should also be treated with standard surgery and chemotherapy, but consideration should be given to single-agent carboplatin until delivery. Given the poorer prognosis of this condition, strong consideration of therapeutic abortion should be discussed with the patient.

Delivery should usually be done by cesarean section, to avoid tumor rupture and fetal dystocia and to perform an optimal staging procedure if it could not be done during the pregnancy. Contrarily to placental choriocarcinoma, which rarely could spread to the embryo, ovarian tumors do not spread to the fetus.

## References

[1] Grimes WH, Bartholomew RA, Colvin ED, et al. Ovarian cyst complicating pregnancy. Am J Obstet Gynecol 1954;68:594–605.
[2] Struyk APHB, Treffers PE. Ovarian tumors in pregnancy. Acta Obstet Gynecol Scand 1984; 63:421–4.
[3] Booth RT. Ovarian tumors in pregnancy. Obstet Gynecol 1963;21:189–92.
[4] White KC. Ovarian tumors in pregnancy. Am J Obstet Gynecol 1973;116:544–50.
[5] Buttery BW, Beisher NA, Fortune DW, et al. Ovarian tumors in pregnancy. Med J Aust 1973;1:345–9.

[6]  Hess W, Peaceman A, O'Brien WF, et al. Adnexal mass occurring with intrauterine pregnancy: report of fifty-four patients requiring laparotomy for definitive management. Am J Obstet Gynecol 1988;158:1029–34.

[7]  Thornton JG, Wells M. Ovarian cysts in pregnancy: does ultrasound make traditional management inappropriate? Obstet Gynecol 1987;69:717–21.

[8]  Tawa K. Ovarian tumors in pregnancy. Am J Obstet Gynecol 1964;90:511–5.

[9]  Hill LM, Johnson CE, Raymond AL. Ovarian surgery in pregnancy. Am J Obstet Gynecol 1975;122:565–9.

[10] Hasan A, Amr S, Issa A, et al. Ovarian tumors complicating pregnancy. Int J Gynaecol Obstet 1983;21:279–82.

[11] Ballard CA. Ovarian tumors associated with pregnancy termination patients. Am J Obstet Gynecol 1984;149:384–7.

[12] Hopkins MP, Duchon MA. Adnexal surgery in pregnancy. J Reprod Med 1986;31:1035–7.

[13] Nelson MJ, Cavalieri R, Graham D, et al. Cysts in pregnancy discovered by sonography. J Clin Ultrasound 1986;14:509–12.

[14] Ashkenazy M, Kessler I, Czernobilsky B, et al. Ovarian tumors in pregnancy. Int J Gynaecol Obstet 1988;27:79–83.

[15] Tchabo JG, Stay EJ, Limaye NS. Ovarian tumors in pregnancy: a community hospital's five year experience. Int Surg 1987;72:227–9.

[16] Koonings PP, Platt LD, Wallace R. Incidental adnexal neoplasms at cesarean section. Obstet Gynecol 1988;72:767–9.

[17] Sunoo CS, Terada KY, Kamemoto LE, et al. Adnexal masses in pregnancy: occurrence by ethnic group. Obstet Gynecol 1990;75:38–40.

[18] El-Yahia AR, Rahman J, Rahman MS, et al. Ovarian tumours in pregnancy. Aust N Z J Obstet Gynaecol 1991;31:327–30.

[19] Platek DN, Henderson CE, Goldberg GL. The management of a persistent mass in pregnancy. Am J Obstet Gynecol 1995;173:1236–40.

[20] Ueda M, Ueki M. Ovarian tumors associated with pregnancy. Int J Gynaecol Obstet 1996;55: 59–65.

[21] Bromley B, Benacerraf B. Adnexal masses during pregnancy: accuracy of sonographic diagnosis and outcome. J Ultrasound Med 1997;16:447–52.

[22] Whitecar MP, Turner S, Higby MK. Adnexal masses in pregnancy: a review of 130 cases undergoing surgical management. Am J Obstet Gynecol 1999;181:19–24.

[23] Oehler M, Wain G, Brand A. Gynaecological malignancies in pregnancy: a review. Aust N Z J Obstet Gynaecol 2003;43:414–20.

[24] Jubb ED. Primary ovarian carcinoma in pregnancy. Am J Obstet Gynecol 1963;85:345–54.

[25] Creasman WT, Rutledge F, Smith JP. Carcinoma of the ovary associated with pregnancy. Obstet Gynecol 1971;38:111–6.

[26] Curtis M, Hopkins MP, Zarlingo T, et al. Magnetic resonance imaging to avoid laparotomy in pregnancy. Obstet Gynecol 1993;82:833–6.

[27] Chiang G, Levine D. Imaging of adnexal masses in pregnancy. J Ultrasound Med 2004; 23:805–19.

[28] Copeland LJ, Landon MB. Malignant disease in pregnancy. In: Gabbe SG, Niebyl JR, Simpson JL, editors. Obstetrics, normal and problem pregnancies. 3rd edition. New York: Churchill Livingstone; 1996. p. 1155–81.

[29] Zalel Y, Piura B, Elchalal U, et al. Diagnosis and management of malignant germ cell ovarian tumors in young females. Int J Gynaecol Obstet 1996;55:1–10.

[30] Talerman A. Germ cell tumours of the ovary. In: Kurman RJ, editor. Blaustein's pathology of the female genital tract. New York: Springer Verlag; 1994. p. 849.

[31] Kumar V, Fausto N, Abbas A. Pathologic basis of disease. 7th edition. St. Louis, Missouri: W.B. Saunders/Elsevier; 2005.

[32] DiSaia PJ, Creasman WT. Clinical gynecologic oncology. 6th edition. St. Louis, Missouri: Mosby; 2002.

[33] Schwartz PE, Morris JM. Serum lactic dehydrogenase: a tumor marker for dysgerminoma. Obstet Gynecol 1988;72:511–5.

[34] Levato F, Martinello R, Campobasso C, et al. LDH and LDH isoenzymes in ovarian dysgerminoma. Eur J Gynaecol Oncol 1995;16:212–5.

[35] Karlen JR, Akbari A, Cook WA. Dysgerminoma associated with pregnancy. Obstet Gynecol 1979;53(3):330–5.

[36] Bakri YN, Ezzat A, Akhtar, et al. Malignant germ cell tumors of the ovary: pregnancy considerations. Eur J Obstet Gynecol Reprod Biol 2000;90:87–91.

[37] Sayedur Rahman M, Al-Sibai MH, Rahman J, et al. Ovarian carcinoma associated with pregnancy: a review of 9 cases. Acta Obstet Gynecol Scand 2002;81:260–4.

[38] Buller RE, Darrow V, Manetta A, et al. Conservative surgical management of dysgerminoma concomitant with pregnancy. Obstet Gynecol 1992;79(5 Pt 2):887–90.

[39] He S, Bremme K, Kallner A, et al. Increased concentrations of lactate dehydrogenase in pregnancy with preeclampsia: a predictor of small for gestational age infants. Gynecol Obstet Invest 1995;39:234–8.

[40] Sheiko MC, Hart WR. Ovarian germinoma (dysgerminoma) with elevated serum lactic dehydrogenase: case report and review of literature. Cancer 1982;49:994–8.

[41] Tojo S, Suzuki A, Fujii S, et al. Tumor markers in gynecologic malignancies. Gan No Rinsho 1983;29:678–83.

[42] Dgani R, Shoham Z, Czernobilsky B, et al. Lactic dehydrogenase, alkaline phosphatase and human chorionic gonadotropin in a pure ovarian dysgerminoma. Gynecol Oncol 1988;30:44–50.

[43] Pressley RH, Muntz HG, Falkenberry S, et al. Serum lactic dehydrogenase as a tumor marker in dysgerminoma. Gynecol Oncol 1992;44:281–3.

[44] Fujita M, Inoue M, Tanizawa O, et al. Retrospective review of 41 patients with endodermal sinus tumor of the ovary. Int J Gynecol Cancer 1993;3:329–35.

[45] Talerman A, Haije G, Baggerman L. Serum alphafetoprotein (AFP) in diagnosis and management of endodermal sinus (yolk sac) tumor and mixed germ cell tumor of the ovary. Cancer 1978;41:272–8.

[46] Weed JC, Roh RA, Mendenhall HW. Recurrent endodermal sinus tumor during pregnancy. Obstet Gynecol 1979;54:653–6.

[47] Petrucha RA, Ruffolo E, Messina AM, et al. Endodermal sinus tumor: report of a case associated with pregnancy. Obstet Gynecol 1980;55(3 Suppl):90S–3S.

[48] Schwartz RP, Chatwani AJ, Strimel W, et al. Endodermal sinus tumor in pregnancy: report of a case and review of the literature. Gynecol Oncol 1983;15:434–9.

[49] Ito K, Teshima K, Suzuki H, et al. A case of ovarian endodermal sinus tumor associated with pregnancy. Tohoku J Exp Med 1984;142:183–94.

[50] Malone JM, Gershenson DM, Creasy RK, et al. Endodermal sinus tumor of the ovary associated with pregnancy. Obstet Gynecol 1986;68(3 Suppl):86S–9S.

[51] Kim DS, Park MI. Maternal and fetal survival following surgery and chemotherapy of endodermal sinus tumor of the ovary during pregnancy: a case report. Obstet Gynecol 1989;73(3 Pt 2):503–7.

[52] Metz SA, Day TG, Pursell SH. Adjuvant chemotherapy in a pregnant patient with endodermal sinus tumor of the ovary. Gynecol Oncol 1989;32:371–4.

[53] Farahmand S, Marchetti D, Asirwatham J, et al. Ovarian endodermal sinus tumor associated with pregnancy: review of the literature. Gynecol Oncol 1991;41:156–60.

[54] Elit L, Bocking A, Kenyon C, et al. An endodermal sinus tumor diagnosed in pregnancy: case report and review of the literature. Gynecol Oncol 1999;72:123–7.

[55] Malhotra N, Sood M. Endodermal sinus tumor in pregnancy. Gynecol Oncol 2000;78:265–6.

[56] Arima N, Tanimoto A, Hayashi R, et al. Ovarian yolk sac tumor with virilization during pregnancy: immunohistochemical demonstration of Leydig cells as functioning stroma. Pathol Int 2000;50:520–5.

[57] Cyganek A, Ejmocka-Ambroziak A, Wiczynska-Zajac A, et al. Ovarian endodermal sinus tumor associated with pregnancy: a case report. Ginekol Pol 2002;73:408–11.

[58] Shimizu Y, Komiyama S, Kobayashi T, et al. Successful management of endodermal sinus tumor of the ovary associated with pregnancy. Gynecol Oncol 2003;88:447–50.

[59] Han JY, Nava-Ocampo AA, Kim TJ, et al. Pregnancy outcome after prenatal exposure to bleomycin, etoposide and cisplatin for malignant ovarian germ cell tumors: report of 2 cases. Reprod Toxicol 2005;19:557–61.

[60] Kurman RJ, Norris HJ. Endodermal sinus tumor of the ovary: a clinico-pathologic analysis of 71 cases. Cancer 1976;38:2404–19.

[61] Tewari K, Cappuccini F, Disaia PJ, et al. Malignant germ cell tumors of the ovary. Obstet Gynecol 2000;95:128–33.

[62] Low JJH, Perrin LC, Crandon AJ, et al. Conservative surgery to preserve ovarian function in patients with malignant ovarian germ cell tumors: a review of 74 cases. Cancer 2000;89: 391–8.

[63] Linasmita V, Srisupundit S, Wilailak S, et al. Recent management of malignant ovarian germ cell tumors: a study of 34 cases. J Obstet Gynaecol Res 1999;25:315–20.

[64] Williams S, Blessing JA, Liao DS. Adjuvant therapy of ovarian germ cell tumors with cisplatin, etoposide and bleomycin: a trial of the Gynecologic Oncology Group. J Clin Oncol 1994;12: 701–6.

[65] Abu-Rustum N, Aghajanian C. Management of malignant germ cell tumors of the ovary. Semin Oncol 1998;25:235–42.

[66] Glinski S. Embryonal carcinoma of the ovary in pregnancy. Ginekol Pol 1971;42:1355–6.

[67] Cunanan Jr RG, Lippes J, Tancinco PA. Choriocarcinoma of the ovary with coexisting normal pregnancy. Obstet Gynecol 1980;55:669–72.

[68] Horbelt D, Delmore J, Meisel R, et al. Mixed germ cell malignancy of the ovary concurrent with pregnancy. Obstet Gynecol 1994;84(4 Pt 2):662–4.

[69] Christman JE, Teng NN, Lebovic GS, et al. Delivery of a normal infant following cisplatin, vinblastine, and bleomycin (PVB) chemotherapy for malignant teratoma of the ovary during pregnancy. Gynecol Oncol 1990;37:292–5.

[70] Montz FJ, Horenstein J, Platt LD, et al. The diagnosis of immature teratoma by maternal serum alpha-fetoprotein screening. Obstet Gynecol 1989;73(3 Pt 2):522–5.

[71] Frederiksen MC, Casanova L, Schink JC. An elevated maternal serum alpha-fetoprotein leading to the diagnosis of an immature teratoma. Int J Gynaecol Obstet 1991;35:343–6.

[72] Bonazzi C, Peccatori F, Colombo N, et al. Pure ovarian immature teratoma, a unique and curable disease: 10 years' experience of 32 prospectively treated patients. Obstet Gynecol 1994; 84:598–604.

[73] Dark GG, Bower M, Newlands ES, et al. Surveillance policy for stage I ovarian germ cell tumors. J Clin Oncol 1997;15:620–4.

[74] Seidman JD, Russell P, Kurman RJ. Surface epithelial tumors of the ovary. In: Kurman RJ, editor. Blaustein's pathology of the female genital tract. New York: Springer-Verlag; 2002. p. 791–904.

[75] Seidman JD, Kurman RJ. Pathology of ovarian carcinoma. Hematol Oncol Clin North Am 2003;17:909–25.

[76] Malfetano JH, Goldkrand JW. Cis-platinum combination chemotherapy during pregnancy for advanced epithelial ovarian carcinoma. Obstet Gynecol 1990;75:545–7.

[77] King LA, Nevin PC, Williams PP, et al. Treatment of advanced epithelial ovarian carcinoma in pregnancy with cisplatin-based chemotherapy. Gynecol Oncol 1991;41:78–80.

[78] Henderson CE, Elia G, Garfinkel D, et al. Platinum chemotherapy during pregnancy for serous cystadenocarcinoma of the ovary. Gynecol Oncol 1993;49:92–4.

[79] Bayhan G, Aban M, Yayla M, et al. Cis-platinum combination chemotherapy during pregnancy for mucinous cystadenocarcinoma of the ovary: case report. Eur J Gynaecol Oncol 1999;20: 231–2.

[80] Ohara N, Teramoto K. Successful treatment of an advanced ovarian serous cystadenocarcinoma

in pregnancy with cisplatin, Adriamycin and cyclophosphamide (CAP) regimen: case report. Clin Exp Obstet Gynecol 2000;27:123–4.

[81] Sood AK, Shahin MS, Soroski JI. Paclitaxel and platinum chemotherapy for ovarian carcinoma during pregnancy. Gynecol Oncol 2001;83:599–600.

[82] Otton G, Higgins S, Phillips KA, et al. A case of early stage epithelial ovarian cancer in pregnancy. Int J Gynecol Cancer 2001;11:413–7.

[83] Mendez LE, Mueller A, Salom E, et al. Paclitaxel and carboplatin chemotherapy administered during pregnancy for advanced epithelial ovarian cancer. Obstet Gynecol 2003;5:1200–2.

[84] Picone O, Lhommé C, Tournaire M, et al. Preservation of pregnancy in a patient with a stage IIIB ovarian epithelial carcinoma diagnosed at 22 weeks of gestation and treated with initial chemotherapy: case report and literature review. Gynecol Oncol 2004;94:600–4.

[85] Kobayashi F, Sagawa N, Nakamura K, et al. Mechanism and clinical significance of elevated CA 125 levels in the sera of pregnant women. Am J Obstet Gynecol 1989;160:563–6.

[86] Fiegler P, Kaminski K, Wegrzyn P. Serum levels of CA-125 antigen during the first trimester of pregnancy complications and the risk of miscarriage. Ginekol Pol 2003;74:345–9.

[87] Fiegler P, Katz M, Kaminski K, et al. Clinical value of a single serum CA-125 level in women with symptoms of imminent abortion during the first trimester of pregnancy. J Reprod Med 2003;48:982–8.

[88] Russell P. Surface epithelial-stromal tumors of the ovary. In: Kurman RJ, editor. Blaustein's pathology of the female genital tract. 4th edition. New York: Springer Verlag; 1994. p. 705.

[89] Morice P, Camatte S, Wicart-Poque F, et al. Results of conservative management of epithelial malignant and borderline ovarian tumours. Hum Reprod Update 2003;9:185–92.

[90] Bell DA, Weinstock MA, Scully RE. Peritoneal implants of ovarian serous borderline tumors: histologic features and prognosis. Cancer 1999;62:2212–22.

[91] Ochiai K, Shinozaki H, Takada A, et al. A retrospective study of 1069 epithelial borderline malignancies of the ovary treated in Japan. Proceedings of the Annual Meeting of the American Society of Clinical Oncology 1998;17:A1429.

[92] International Federation of Gynaecoloy and Obstetrics. Annual report and results of treatment in gynaecologic cancer. Int J Gynecol Obstet 1989;28:189–90.

[93] Trimble E, Kaern J, Tropé C. Management of the borderline tumors of the ovary. In: Gershenson DM, Mcguire WP, editors. Ovarian cancer: controversies in management. New York: Churchill Livingstone; 1998.

[94] Morice P, Camatte S, El Hassan J, et al. Clinical outcomes and fertility results after conservative treatment for ovarian borderline tumor. Fertil Steril 2001;75:92–6.

[95] Lackman F, Carey MS, Kirk ME, et al. Surgery as sole treatment for serous borderline tumors of the ovary with noninvasive implants. Gynecol Oncol 2003;90:407–12.

[96] Gershenson D, Silva E, Levy L, et al. Ovarian serous borderline tumors with invasive peritoneal implants. Cancer 1998;82:1096–103.

[97] Darai E, Teboul J, Walker F, et al. Epithelial ovarian carcinoma of low malignant potential. Eur J Obstet Gynecol Reprod Biol 1996;66:141–5.

[98] Zanetta G, Rota S, Chiari S, et al. Behavior of borderline tumors with particular interest to persistence, recurrence, and progression to invasive carcinoma: a prospective study. J Clin Oncol 2001;19:2658–64.

[99] Camatte S, Rouzier R, Boccara-Dekeyser J, et al. Prognosis and fertility after conservative treatment for ovarian tumors of limited malignity: review of 68 cases. Gynecol Obstet Fertil 2002;30:583–91.

[100] Camatte S, Morice P, Pautier P, et al. Fertility results after conservative treatment of advanced stage serous borderline tumour of the ovary. BJOG 2002;109:376–80.

[101] Barnhill DR, Kurman RJ, Brady MF, et al. Preliminary analysis of the behavior of stage I ovarian serous tumors of low malignant potential: a Gynecologic Oncology Group study. J Clin Oncol 1995;13:2752–6.

[102] Zanetta G, Chiari S, Rota S, et al. Conservative surgery for stage I ovarian carcinoma in women of childbearing age. Br J Obstet Gynaecol 1997;104:1030–5.

[103] Lim-Tan SK, Cajigas HE, Scully RE. Ovarian cystectomy for serous borderline tumors: a follow-up study of 35 cases. Obstet Gynecol 1998;72:775–81.

[104] Darai E, Teboul J, Fauconnier A, et al. Management and outcome of borderline ovarian tumors incidentally discovered at or after laparoscopy. Acta Obstet Gynecol Scand 1998;77:451–7.

[105] Trope CG, Kristensen G, Makar M. Surgery for borderline tumor of the ovary. Semin Surg Oncol 2000;19:69–75.

[106] Donnez J, Munschke A, Berliere M, et al. Safety of conservative management and fertility outcome in women with borderline tumors of the ovary. Fertil Steril 2003;79:1216–21.

[107] Fauvet R, Poncelet C, Boccara J, et al. Fertility after conservative treatment for borderline ovarian tumors: a French multicenter study. Fertil Steril 2005;83:284–90.

[108] Wang PH, Chao HT, Too LL, et al. Borderline ovarian tumors complicating pregnancy: a case report. Zhonghua Yi Xue Za Zhi (Taipei) 1999;62:179–83.

[109] Studzinski Z, Filipczak A, Branicka D. Coexistence of ovarian epithelial tumor of borderline malignancy with pregnancy: a case report. Ginekol Pol 1999;70:101–4.

[110] Mikami M, Ono A, Sakaiya N, et al. Case report of serous ovarian tumor of borderline malignancy (stage Ic) in a pregnant woman. Eur J Obstet Gynecol Reprod Biol 2001;98:237–9.

[111] Fort MG, Pierce VK, Saigo PE, et al. Evidence of the efficacy of adjuvant chemotherapy in epithelial ovarian tumors of low malignant potential. Gynecol Oncol 1989;32:269–72.

[112] Barakat RR, Benjamin IB, Lewis Jr JL, et al. Platinum-based chemotherapy for advanced-stage serous ovarian cancers of low malignant potential. Gynecol Oncol 1990;59:390–5.

[113] Gershenson DM, Silva EG. Serous ovarian tumors of low malignant potential with peritoneal implants. Cancer 1990;65:578–85.

[114] Makar AP, Kaern J, Kristensen GB, et al. Evaluation of serum CA 125 level as a tumor marker in borderline tumors of the ovary. Int J Gynecol Cancer 1993;3:299–303.

[115] Kaern J, Trope CG, Abeler VM. A retrospective study of 370 borderline tumors of the ovary treated at the Norwegian Radium Hospital from 1970 to 1982: a review of clinicopathologic features and treatment modalities. Cancer 1993;71:1810–20.

[116] Seracchioli R, Venturoli S, Colombo FM, et al. Fertility and tumor recurrence rate after conservative laparoscopic management of young women with early-stage borderline ovarian tumors. Fertil Steril 2001;76:999–1004.

[117] Camatte S, Morice P, Pautier P, et al. Fertility results after conservative treatment of advanced stage serous borderline tumour of the ovary. BJOG 2002;109:376–80.

[118] Donnez J, Munschke A, Berliere M, et al. Safety of conservative management and fertility outcome in women with borderline tumors of the ovary. Fertil Steril 2003;79:1216–21.

[119] Young R, Clement PB, Scully RE. The ovary. In: Sternberg SS, editor. Diagnostic surgical pathology. New York: Raven Press; 1989. p. 116–31.

[120] Robertson DM, Stephenson T, Pruysers E, et al. Inhibins/activins as diagnostic markers for ovarian cancer. Mol Cell Endocrinol 2002;191:97–103.

[121] Jaworski RC, Fryatt JJ, Turner TB, et al. Gynandroblastoma of the ovary. Pathology 1986;18: 348–51.

[122] Fukunaga M, Endo Y, Ushigome S. Gynandroblastoma of the ovary: a case report with an immunohistochemical and ultrastructural study. Virchows Arch 1997;430:77–82.

[123] Young RH, Scully RE. Ovarian Sertoli-Leydig cell tumors: a clinicopathological analysis of 207 cases. Am J Surg Pathol 1985;9:543–69.

[124] Horny HP, Braumann W, Weiss E, et al. Virilizing stromal Leydig cell tumor (Leydig cell-containing thecoma) of the ovary in pregnancy: a case report with extensive immunohistochemical investigation of the tumor cells. Gen Diagn Pathol 1995;141:57–60.

[125] Fox H, Agrawal K, Langley FA. A clinicopathologic study of 92 cases of granulosa cell tumor of the ovary with special reference to the factors influencing prognosis. Cancer 1975;35: 231–41.

[126] Pankratz E, Boyes DA, White GW, et al. Granulosa cell tumors: a clinical review of 61 cases. Obstet Gynecol 1978;52:718–23.

[127] Stenwig JT, Hazekamp JT, Beecham JB. Granulosa cell tumors of the ovary: a clinicopathological study of 118 cases with long-term follow up. Gynecol Oncol 1979;7:136–52.

[128] Evans AT, Gaffey TA, Malkasian GD, et al. Clinicopathologic review of 118 granulosa and 82 theca cell tumors. Obstet Gynecol 1980;55:231 – 8.

[129] Ohel G, Kaneti H, Schenker JG. Granulosa cell tumors in Israel: a study of 172 cases. Gynecol Oncol 1983;15:278 – 86.

[130] Schumer ST, Cannistra SA. Granulosa cell tumor of the ovary. J Clin Oncol 2003;21:1180 – 9.

[131] Zaloudek C, Norris HJ. Sertoli-Leydig tumors of the ovary: a clinicopathologic study of 64 intermediate and poorly differentiated neoplasms. Am J Surg Pathol 1984;8:405 – 18.

[132] Young RH, Dudley AG, Scully RE. Granulosa cell, Sertoli-Leydig cell, and unclassified sex cord-stromal tumors associated with pregnancy: a clinicopathological analysis of thirty-six cases. Gynecol Oncol 1984;18:181 – 205.

[133] Kalir T, Friedman Jr F. Gynandroblastoma in pregnancy: case report and review of literature. Mt Sinai J Med 1998;65:292 – 5.

[134] Tomlinson MW, Treadwell MC, Deppe G. Platinum based chemotherapy to treat recurrent Sertoli-Leydig cell ovarian carcinoma during pregnancy. Eur J Gynaecol Oncol 1997;18:44 – 6.

[135] Williams SD, Birch R, Einhorn LH, et al. Treatment of disseminated germ-cell tumors with cisplatin, bleomycin, and either vinblastine or etoposide. N Engl J Med 1987;316:1435 – 40.

[136] Gershenson DM, Morris M, Burke TW, et al. Treatment of poor prognosis sex-cord stromal tumors of the ovary with the combination of bleomycin, etoposide, and cisplatin. Obstet Gynecol 1996;87:527 – 31.

[137] Savage P, Constenla D, Fisher C, et al. Granulosa cell tumors of the ovary: demographics, survival and the management of advanced disease. Clin Oncol (R Coll Radiol) 1998;10:242 – 5.

[138] Homesley HD, Bundy BN, Hurteau JA, et al. Bleomycin, etoposide and cisplatin combination therapy of ovarian granulosa cell tumors and other stromal malignancies: a Gynecologic Oncology Group study. Gynecol Oncol 1999;72:131 – 7.

[139] Clement PB. Tumor-like lesions of the ovary associated with pregnancy. Int J Gynecol Pathol 1993;12:108 – 15.

[140] Boggess JF, Soules MR, Goff BA, et al. Serum inhibin and disease status in women with ovarian granulosa cell tumors. Gynecol Oncol 1997;64:64 – 9.

[141] Jobling T, Mamers P, Healy DL, et al. A prospective study of inhibin in granulosa cell tumors of the ovary. Gynecol Oncol 1994;55:285 – 9.

[142] Healy DL, Burger HG, Mamers P, et al. Elevated serum inhibin concentrations in post-menopausal women with ovarian tumors. N Engl J Med 1993;329:1539 – 42.

[143] Rey RA, Lhomme C, Marcillac I, et al. Antimullerian hormone as a serum marker of granulosa cell tumors of the ovary: comparative study with serum alpha-inhibin and estradiol. Am J Obstet Gynecol 1996;174:958 – 65.

[144] Lane AH, Lee MM, Fuller Jr AF, et al. Diagnostic utility of mullerian inhibiting substance determination in patients with primary and recurrent granulosa cell tumors. Gynecol Oncol 1999;73:51 – 5.

[145] Hernandez W, DiSaia PJ, Morrow CP, et al. Mixed mesodermal sarcoma of the ovary. Obstet Gynecol 1999;49(Suppl 1):59 – 63.

[146] Hanjani P, Petersen RO, Lipton SE, et al. Malignant mixed mesodermal tumors and carcino-sarcoma of the ovary: report of eight cases and review of the literature. Obstet Gynecol Surv 1983;38:537 – 45.

[147] DiSilvestro PA, Gajewski WH, Ludwig ME, et al. Malignant mixed mesodermal tumors of the ovary. Obstet Gynecol 1995;86:780 – 2.

[148] Kowalski MS. Case of primary sarcoma of the ovary in pregnancy. Pol Tyg Lek (Wars) 1954; 9:12 – 4.

[149] Schroder H. Sarcoma and carcinoma of ovary in pregnancy. Zentralbl Gynakol 1966;88: 1047 – 51.

[150] Bonevat N, Sophonn S, San LK, et al. Ovarian sarcoma and pregnancy (apropos of a personal case). Bull Fed Soc Gynecol Obstet Lang Fr 1967;19:214 – 5.

[151] As AK, Webb JB, Chowdhury RR. Malignant mixed mesodermal tumour of the ovary: clinicopathological features. J Obstet Gynaecol 1999;19:643 – 6.

[152] Morrow CP, d'Ablaing G, Brady LW, et al. A clinical and pathologic study of 30 cases of malignant mixed mullerian epithelial and mesenchymal ovarian tumors: a Gynecologic Oncology Group study. Gynecol Oncol 1984;18:278–92.

[153] Piura B, Rabinovich A, Yanai-Inbar I, et al. Primary sarcoma of the ovary: report of five cases and review of the literature. Eur J Gynaecol Oncol 1998;19:257–61.

[154] Barwick KW, LiVolsi VA. Malignant mixed mesodermal tumors of the ovary: a clinicopathologic assessment of 12 cases. Am J Surg Pathol 1980;4:37–42.

[155] Brown E, Stewart M, Rye T, et al. Carcinosarcoma of the ovary: 19 years of prospective data from a single center. Cancer 2004;100:2148–53.

[156] Le T, Krepart GV, Lotocki RJ, et al. Malignant mixed mesodermal ovarian tumor treatment and prognosis: a 20-year experience. Gynecol Oncol 1997;65:237–40.

[157] Simon SR, Wang SE, Uhl M, et al. Complete response of carcinosarcoma of the ovary to therapy with doxorubicin, ifosfamide, and dacarbazine. Gynecol Oncol 1991;41:161–6.

[158] Patsner B, Greenberg S. Mesna, doxorubicin, ifosfamide, and dacarbazine chemotherapy for ovarian mixed mullerian sarcoma: report of four cases. Gynecol Oncol 1995;58:386–8.

[159] Yada-Hashimoto N, Yamamoto T, Kamiura S, et al. Metastatic ovarian tumors: a review of 64 cases. Gynecol Oncol 2003;89:314–7.

[160] Mandai M, Konishi I, Tsuruta Y, et al. Krukenberg tumor from an occult appendiceal adenocarcinoid: a case report and review of the literature. Eur J Obstet Gynecol Reprod Biol 2001;97:90–5.

[161] Tebeu PM, Pelte MF, Anguenot JL, et al. Krukenberg tumour from an appendiceal carcinoma presenting as a primary ovarian tumour. West Indian Med J 2004;53:427–8.

[162] Robboy SJ, Scully RE, Norris HJ. Carcinoid metastatic to the ovary: a clinicopathologic analysis of 35 cases. Cancer 1974;33:798–811.

[163] Kuhlman JE, Hruban RH, Fishman EK. Krukenberg tumors: CT features and growth characteristics. South Med J 1989;82:1215–9.

[164] Kasahara A, Nagakura T, Oshita M, et al. A case with goblet cell carcinoid of the appendix presenting as unilateral Krukenberg tumor. Nippon Shokakibyo Gakkai Zasshi 1991;88:1474–8.

[165] Loke TK, Lo SS, Chan CS. Case report: Krukenberg tumours arising from a primary duodenojejunal adenocarcinoma. Clin Radiol 1997;52:154–5.

[166] Prat J. Ovarian carcinomas, including secondary tumors: diagnostically challenging areas. Mod Pathol 2005;18(Suppl 2):S99–111.

[167] Robboy SJ, Norris HJ, Scully RE. Insular carcinoid primary in the ovary: a clinicopathologic analysis of 48 cases. Cancer 1975;36:404–18.

[168] Fox H, Langley FA, Govan AD, et al. Malignant lymphoma presenting as an ovarian tumour: a clinicopathological analysis of 34 cases. Br J Obstet Gynaecol 1988;95:386–90.

[169] Monterroso V, Jaffe ES, Merino MJ, et al. Malignant lymphomas involving the ovary: a clinicopathologic analysis of 39 cases. Am J Surg Pathol 1993;17:154–70.

[170] Miannay E, Detourmignies L, Decocq J, et al. Malignant non-Hodgkins lymphoma manifested in an ovarian tumor: five case reports. J Gynecol Obstet Biol Reprod (Paris) 1997;26:424–9.

[171] Baloglu H, Turken O, Tutuncu L, et al. 24-year-old female with amenorrhea: bilateral primary ovarian Burkitt lymphoma. Gynecol Oncol 2003;91:449–51.

[172] Parry-Jones E. Krukenberg tumour complicating pregnancy. J Obstet Gynaecol Br Emp 1956;63:592–3.

[173] Lawrence WD, Larson PN, Hauge ET. Primary Krukenberg tumor of the ovary in pregnancy: report of a case; discussion. Obstet Gynecol 1957;10:84–8.

[174] Braga AI, Ferreira A. Krukenberg tumor and pregnancy. Rev Med Aeron Braz 1958;10:90–101.

[175] Alwyn JE, Zacharin RF. Pregnancy complicated by torsion of a unilateral Krukenberg tumour. Aust N Z J Obstet Gynaecol 1963;41:125–8.

[176] Sonnino S, Caporale F. Krukenberg tumor and pregnancy. Riv Obstet Ginecol 1963;18:353–61.

[177] Engeler V, Siebenmann R, Schreiner WE. Primary Krukenberg tumour in pregnancy. Arch Gynakol 1976;220:293–300.

[178] Sedgely MG, Ostor AG, Fortune DW. Angiosarcoma of breast metastatic to the ovary and placenta. Aust N Z J Obstet Gynaecol 1985;25:299–302.

[179] Choudhary S. Krukenberg tumour associated with pregnancy. J Indian Med Assoc 1986;84: 56–7.

[180] Yakushiji M, Tazaki T, Nishimura H, et al. Krukenberg tumors of the ovary: a clinicopathologic analysis of 112 cases. Nippon Sanka Fujinka Gakkai Zasshi 1987;39:479–85.

[181] Cheng CY, Chen TY, Lin CK, et al. Krukenberg tumor in pregnancy with delivery of a normal baby: a case report. Zhonghua Yi Xue Za Zhi (Taipei) 1994;54:424–7.

[182] Tamussino K, Scholl W, Reich O, et al. Gastric carcinoma presenting as a Krukenberg tumor in the 24th week of gestation. Eur J Obstet Gynecol Reprod Biol 1995;62:251–2.

[183] Mackey JR, Hugh J, Smylie M. Krukenberg tumor complicated by pregnancy. Gynecol Oncol 1996;61:153–5.

[184] Sandmeier D, Lobrinus JA, Vial Y, et al. Bilateral Krukenberg tumor of the ovary during pregnancy. Eur J Gynaecol Oncol 2000;21:58–60.

[185] Cosme A, Ojeda E, Bujanda L, et al. Krukenberg tumor secondary to gastric carcinoma in a woman in her eighth month of pregnancy. Gastroenterol Hepatol 2001;24:63–5.

[186] Agarwal N, Parul, Kriplani A, et al. Management and outcome of pregnancies complicated with adnexal masses. Arch Gynecol Obstet 2003;267:148–52.

[187] Ulbright TM, Roth LM, Stehman FB. Secondary ovarian neoplasia: a clinicopathologic study of 35 cases. Cancer 1984;5:1164–74.

[188] Lash RH, Hart WR. Intestinal adenocarcinomas metastatic to the ovaries: a clinicopathologic evaluation of 22 cases. Am J Surg Pathol 1987;11:114–21.

[189] Bell RJ. Fetal virilisation due to maternal Krukenberg tumor. Lancet 1977;1:1162–3.

[190] Vicens E, Martinez-Mora J, Potau N, et al. Masculinization of a female fetus by Krukenberg tumor during pregnancy. J Pediatr Surg 1980;15:188–90.

[191] Silva PD, Porto M, Moyer DL, et al. Clinical and ultrastructural findings of an androgenizing Krukenberg tumor in pregnancy. Obstet Gynecol 1988;71(3 Pt 2):432–4.

[192] Fung MF, Vadas G, Lotocki R, et al. Tubular Krukenberg tumor in pregnancy with virilization. Gynecol Oncol 1991;41:81–4.

[193] Spadoni LR, Lindberg MC, Mottet NK, et al. Virilization coexisting with Krukenberg tumor during pregnancy. Am J Obstet Gynecol 1965;92:981–91.

[194] de Palma P, Wronski M, Bifernino V, et al. Krukenberg tumor in pregnancy with virilization: a case report. Eur J Gynaecol Oncol 1995;16:59–64.

[195] Vauthier-Brouzes D, Vanna Lim-You K, Sebagh E, et al. Krukenberg tumor during pregnancy with maternal and fetal virilization: a difficult diagnosis: a case report. Gynecol Obstet Biol Reprod (Paris) 1997;26:831–3.

[196] Scully RE, Young RH, Clement PB. Tumors of the ovary, maldeveloped gonads, fallopian tube, and broad ligament. In: Atlas of tumor pathology, Third Series, Fascicle 23. Washington: AFIP; 1998. p. 81–105.

ELSEVIER
SAUNDERS

Obstet Gynecol Clin N Am
32 (2005) 595–614

OBSTETRICS AND
GYNECOLOGY
CLINICS
OF NORTH AMERICA

# Hematologic Malignancies in Pregnancy

Timothy J. Hurley, MD[a,b,*], James V. McKinnell, MD[c],
Mehraboon S. Irani, MD[d]

[a]Division of Maternal and Fetal Medicine, Department of Obstetrics and Gynecology,
University of New Mexico Health Science Center, 2211 Lomas Boulevard,
Albuquerque, NM 87131, USA
[b]The Mother Baby Unit, University of New Mexico Health Science Center, 2211 Lomas Boulevard,
Albuquerque, NM 87131, USA
[c]Division of Oncology and Haematology, Department of Pediatrics,
University of New Mexico Health Science Center, MSC10-5590, 1 University of New Mexico,
Albuquerque, NM 87131, USA
[d]Division of Haematology, Department of Pathology, Presbyterian Hospital, Tricore Laboratory,
1100 Central Avenue, Albuquerque, NM 87106, USA

Hematologic malignances, as a group, represent 25% of the cancers complicating pregnancy, behind carcinomas of the breast (26%) and cancer of the uterine cervix (26%) [1–3]. In women 15 to 24 years of age, however, the most frequent malignant tumor is Hodgkin's lymphoma (HL) [4]. Like other cancers complicating pregnancy, they are uncommon, with the incidence of HL during gestation reported at 1:1000 to 1:6000, whereas the incidence of leukemia coincident with pregnancy is reported at 1:75,000 to 1:100,000 [1–3]. Clearly, no single individual can have sufficient experience with these malignancies to be considered an expert. It is imperative that a multidisciplinary team involving oncologists, pediatric specialists, nurse coordinators, and obstetricians care for patients with hematologic malignancies. The primary role of the obstetrician is to assist in the diagnosis of these disorders and to coordinate the various subspecialty consultations. The obstetrician should also play an integral role in counseling the patient and her family regarding their options and establishing the timing and method of delivery.

* Corresponding author. Division of Maternal and Fetal Medicine, Department of Obstetrics and Gynecology, University of New Mexico Health Science Center, 2211 Lomas Boulevard, Albuquerque, NM 87131.
E-mail address: thurley@salud.unm.edu (T.J. Hurley).

This article discusses the three most common categories of hematologic malignancies: (1) HL, (2) non-Hodgkin's lymphoma (NHL), and (3) leukemia. Case vignettes are used to illustrate the importance of early diagnosis on maternal and fetal prognosis, the effect of the disease on the pregnancy, and the effect of pregnancy on the disease. Finally, the effect of pregnancy on the available treatment options is also discussed.

## Vignette 1: Hodgkin's lymphoma

A 25-year-old white woman, $G_2P_{1001}$, presented for her follow-up prenatal visit at 29 weeks without complaints other than an enlarged nontender mass in her right axilla that had been present for the last 2 months. This finding was thought to represent extramammary tissue, and the patient was reassured and scheduled for a follow-up appointment in 3 weeks. At the patient's follow-up appointment, it was believed that the mass was more enlarged, measuring 3 × 3 cm, firm and nontender. There was no history of night sweats, fever, or weight loss, but she did complain of increased pruritus over the last few weeks. She had a history of having mononucleosis, while she was a college student; otherwise, her medical history was unremarkable. Her hemoglobin, hematocrit, leukocyte levels, and platelet count and electrolytes, erythrocyte sedimentation rate, and liver function studies were all normal. Serologies for acute infection with cytomegalovirus, toxoplasmosis, HIV, and her heterophile antibody test were all negative. After referral to a hematologist at 32 weeks, the patient underwent a lymph node biopsy that was histologically classified as HL of nodular sclerosis subtype. Bone marrow biopsy was negative. Chest and abdominal MRI showed some mediastinal enlargement (<10 cm), but no evidence of abdominal para-aortic lymph node enlargement, hepatic or spleen enlargement, or occult bone marrow involvement.

Based on these results the patient was staged as clinical stage 1A and her treatment options were discussed. She and her family elected to delay treatment until after delivery. Antenatal steroids were administered and her labor was induced after fetal lung maturation was confirmed at 35 weeks. Both the patient and infant did well and were discharged home on postpartum day 2. The patient was scheduled for follow-up with oncology for further treatment.

## Hodgkin's lymphoma

HL is a disease of young adults with an average age of diagnosis in pregnant and nonpregnant women of 25.5 years [5]. It accounts for 51% of the hematologic malignancies complicating pregnancy and is the fourth most common cancer encountered during gestation [1–3]. HL is a neoplasm that originates in the lymph nodes and seems to spread contiguously from one lymph node group to another. It often presents with painless lymphadenopathy, usually of the

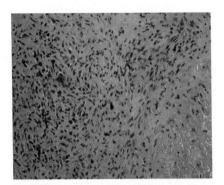

Fig. 1. Hodgkin lymphoma, nodular sclerosis type, showing sclerosis with lymphocytes, histiocytes, and a multinucleated Reed-Sternberg cell (*left center*). Necrosis is also present (*lower right*), which may be seen in this type of lymphoma (hematoxylin-eosin, original magnification ×100).

cervical, submaxillary, or axillary nodes. The etiology is uncertain, but is probably multifactorial with both a genetic predisposition (based on studies of familial aggregation) and environmental factors (based on the finding of Epstein-Barr virus DNA) in up to 50% of biopsy specimens [6]. HL is a pathologic diagnosis, characterized by the presence of the clonal malignant Hodgkin cell or multinucleated Reed-Sternberg cell in a background mixture of reactive, inflammatory, and stromal cells (Figs. 1 and 2). Until the mid-late 1990s, the origin of the Reed-Sternberg cell was obscure. It has recently been demonstrated, however, that these cells are of B-cell lineage [7]. These tumors can be subclassified based on their histopathologic characteristics (World Health Organization [WHO] classification), with the most common histologic subtype, nodular sclerosis, also occurring most frequently in pregnancy. In the past, the histologic subtype was believed to have important prognostic significance, with the nodular sclerosis subtype conferring a more favorable prognosis. More recently, however, with advancements in the treatment of HL, the two most important and consistent prognostic factors that have emerged are the stage of disease (modified Ann

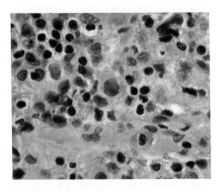

Fig. 2. Multinucleated Reed-Sternberg cell (*center*) with surrounding benign lymphocytes and histiocytes, in the same patient as Fig. 1 (hematoxylin-eosin, original magnification ×400).

Arbor system for staging) and the patient's age. Patients who are less than 60 years of age and who have limited-stage disease can expect long-term survival rates of at least 90% [8]. The Ann Arbor staging system incorporates the number and location of involved lymph nodes, the presence of extralymphatic extensions, and the presence or absence of B symptoms (unexplained weight loss, recurrent fever >38°C, and recurrent night sweats) into a prognostically valuable system for staging lymphomas [9]. In North America, patients with Ann Arbor stage I to II, the absence of bulky disease (tumor mass <10 cm), and without B symptoms are considered to have early stage disease [10].

Pregnancy itself does not seem to affect the stage of the disease at diagnosis, the response to therapy, or the overall survival rate when compared with age- and stage-equivalent nonpregnant controls [11,12]. In addition, pregnancy termination does not seem to improve maternal outcome. Approximately 70% of pregnant patients with HL present with early stage disease (stage I–II) with 8-year survival rates of 83% [4,11]. In the past, staging for HL was both clinical and pathologic, with pathologic staging accomplished by laparotomy. With the use of modern-generation CT and MRI studies, however, and current multiagent chemotherapeutic regimens of doxorubicin, bleomycin, vinblastine, and dacarbazine, the need for staging laparotomy is uncommon [10].

The initial evaluation should include a complete history and physical with careful documentation of B-symptoms. In addition, a thorough documentation of all node-bearing areas should be performed. A complete differential blood count and platelets, an erythrocyte sedimentation rate, tests for liver and renal function, and assays for lactate dehydrogenase and alkaline phosphatase should be obtained. Radiologic studies should include a chest radiograph and an MRI of the chest, abdomen, and pelvis. Although usually negative, bone marrow biopsies are recommended. Fortunately, lymphangiograms, which should be avoided during pregnancy because of potential fetal radiation exposure, are rarely used in the current evaluation of HL patients.

Whether or not HL adversely affects pregnancy is less clear. In the studies performed to date, with some of the reported patients opting to delay treatment until after delivery, there does not seem to be a significant difference in birth weight, mean gestational age, or method of delivery [12,13]. In addition, one study was done of 26 mothers with advanced-stage HL, with treatment started in all three trimesters using combined chemotherapy of doxorubicin, bleomycin, vinblastine, and dacarbazine; mechlorethamine, vincristine, prednisone, and procarbazine; or epirubicin, bleomycin, vinblastine, and dacarbazine. The study found no evidence at long-term follow-up (median age, 18.3 years) of congenital anomalies, hematologic malignancies, or neurodevelopmental abnormalities in any of the individuals exposed to these chemotherapeutic agents in utero [13]. Other studies, however, particularly if treatment is started in the first trimester, have been less optimistic, with fetal anomalies, fetal demise, fetal growth restriction, premature deliveries, and neonatal pancytopenia all reported with various, but not necessarily identical, multiagent chemotherapeutic regimens [14,15].

The treatment for early stage HL has undergone a significant metamorphosis over the last decade. In the past, the mainstay of treatment for early stage HL was external-beam radiation therapy, with the mantle field (axillary, cervical, mediastinal, and pulmonary hilar lymph nodes) used for supradiaphragmatic disease. In the early 1990s, to decrease the relapse rate (40%) with radiation therapy alone, and to avoid the morbidity associated with staging laparotomy and the emerging problem of secondary solid malignancies, the use of combined modality therapy was introduced and later refined [16,17]. Clinical trials of combined modality therapy, involving the use of multiagent chemotherapy (doxorubicin, bleomycin, vinblastine, and dacarbazine) plus low-dose involved-field radiotherapy, have produced overall survival rates of 93% [18]. These results have encouraged many experts to recommend, even during pregnancy, that patients with early stage disease be treated with multiagent chemotherapy, preferably doxorubicin, bleomycin, vinblastine, and dacarbazine, with or without involved-field radiotherapy. If involved-field radiotherapy is elected, the study by Woo and coworkers [19] has particular relevance. In this observational study, 11 women with stage IA to IIA nodular sclerosing HL were treated at various gestational ages with mantle irradiation (4000 cGy) doses that far exceed those currently recommended (2800–3200 cGy). Despite these relatively high doses, with proper uterine shielding, the highest estimated fetal dose was 13.6 cGy [19]. Furthermore, none of the infants demonstrated any adverse effects from this exposure. Given that the fetal risks of ionizing radiation are both a gestational age and threshold phenomenon with the risk for congenital malformations, microcephaly, and miscarriage in the first trimester increasing after a dose of 20 cGy, and the threshold dose for mental retardation at 8 to 15 weeks of gestation reported to be 18 cGy, it seems reasonable that treatment in the second and early third trimester for patients with early stage disease should not be altered by the pregnancy [20,21]. In the first trimester, because of concerns for possible adverse fetal effects from multiagent chemotherapy (7%–17%) risk of fetal anomalies, the risk of delaying chemotherapy, progression of maternal disease to a higher stage needs to be balanced with the patient's desire to avoid potential harm to her fetus. In the third trimester, however, there are few circumstances in which radiation therapy is used before delivery can be accomplished. In this situation antenatal steroids should be administered and delivery accomplished after 32 to 34 weeks gestational age, once fetal lung maturation can be confirmed by amniocentesis. If spontaneous labor ensues after 32 weeks it should be allowed to progress, as long as antenatal steroids have been previously administered, and there are no obstetric indications contradicting spontaneous vaginal delivery [22]. Delivery, if possible, should be timed 2 to 3 weeks after chemotherapy, to avoid the maximum risk of neonatal myelosuppression.

Treatment of pregnant patients with advanced-stage disease is best accomplished with multiagent chemotherapy. Long-term disease-free survival rates of 88% have been observed in advanced-stage patients treated with mechlorethamine, vincristine, prednisone, and procarbazine; doxorubicin, bleomycin, vinblastine, and dacarbazine; or epirubicin, bleomycin, vinblastine, and dacarbazine [13].

There is no evidence that method of delivery should be affected by the presence of HL complicating pregnancy. Pathologic examination of the placenta should be considered because placental metastases, although rare, have been documented [2]. In addition, the patient should be counseled regarding the option of cord blood banking as a source of HLA-compatible stem cells [23,24]. Finally, patients who maintain their fertility after treatment should be advised to avoid pregnancy for at least 2 years, because this is the time of greatest risk for relapse after primary therapy [25].

## Vignette 2: non-Hodgkin's lymphoma

The pregnancy of a 38-year-old woman, $G_2P_{1001}$, had been uneventful until 10 days before admission, when she developed a sore throat, nonproductive cough, vomiting, and a fever. At 27 weeks' gestational age, she was hospitalized in advanced labor with a cervix dilated to 5 cm and 100% effaced. She had a temperature of 38.8°C, a pulse of 120 bpm, and the fetal heart rate was 160 bpm. No lymphadenopathy was appreciated and her lung fields were believed to be clear. Ultrasound demonstrated an appropriately grown fetus with normal biophysical profile (BPP) and amniotic fluid volume. There were no fetal or placental abnormalities noted. Laboratory data revealed a white blood cell count of 3800/μL, 39% bands, 25% lymphocytes. Her hematocrit was 40% with normal indices; a platelet count was 130,000/μL. Liver functions demonstrated a serum glutamic-oxaloacetic transaminase of 31 U/L and a lactic dehydrogenase of 1697 U/L. Her initial chest radiograph demonstrated a left lower lobe infiltrate and she was started on broad-spectrum parenteral antibiotics.

She progressed rapidly and delivered a 1.214-g girl vaginally, with Apgar scores of 4 and 5. She suffered an immediate postpartum hemorrhage that required manual extraction of the placenta and curettage, and uterotonic to control. The placenta was noted to be friable but was not sent for pathologic investigation. On the evening of her first postpartum day she became tachypneic and her temperature rose to 39°C. Her chest radiograph revealed bilateral pleural effusions. Repeat complete blood count demonstrated a white blood count of 4800/μL; hematocrit of 27%; platelet count of 88,000/μL; prothrombin time 14.8 seconds (control 13 seconds); partial thromboplastin time 63 seconds (control 30 seconds); and a fibrinogen of 103 mg/dL. The patient ultimately required mechanical ventilation for worsening hypoxia and acidosis. Despite aggressive treatment with vasopressors, antibiotics, and blood products, her condition continued to deteriorate and she expired on the fourth postpartum day.

Examination of the patient at necropsy revealed severe pulmonary edema, hepatosplenomegaly but no lymphadenopathy. Microscopic examination of the liver revealed lymphoid infiltrates comprised of mitotically active large lymphoid cells. Cellular infiltrates of similar appearance were present in the uterine myometrium, ovaries, spleen, and the perivascular tissue of the lung. Lymph nodes and bone marrow, however, were not involved. Immunohistochemical studies of paraffin-imbedded tissue from the liver and myometrium were positive for CD 43 and negative for CD 30, CD 20, and Ki-M1P. These histologic and immunologic features were consistent with a non-Hodgkin's T-cell lymphoma that would now probably be classified as a hepatosplenic T-cell lymphoma (WHO classification).

The infant's initial course was unremarkable; however, at 2 months of age she developed respiratory distress and required intubation. An open lung biopsy demonstrated perivascular large mitotically active lymphoid infiltrates, which were cytologically identical to those present in the mother. Immunohistochemistry revealed a cell phenotype identical to that found in the mother's tissues.

The infant was started on induction chemotherapy with cyclophosphamide, doxorubicin, etoposide, and prednisone. In addition, intrathecal treatment with methotrexate, arabinosylcytosine, and hydrocortisone was initiated. She entered remission and was placed on maintenance chemotherapy for 1 year and has remained in complete remission [5].

## Non-Hodgkin's lymphoma

The NHLs are a heterogeneous group of lymphoid malignancies that have their origins in lymphoreticular tissue. They are separated from HL by the absence of Reed-Sternberg cells. NHLs are tumors of either T- or B-cell origin and differ in their presentation, stage at diagnosis, and prognosis. Some follow an indolent course, with small component cells and retention of a follicular architecture, whereas others are aggressive tumors with primitive blasts and loss of the normal nodal structure (Fig. 3). Approximately 88% of NHLs are derived from monoclonal populations of B cells [26]. In pregnancy and patients younger than 35 years of age, however, there seems to be a disproportionate number of T-cell and indeterminate phenotypes [27,28].

Unlike HL, which has its peak incidence in the reproductive years, NHL occurs with a mean age at diagnosis of 42 years. The estimated incidence during

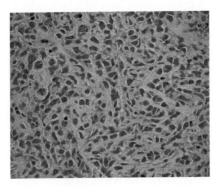

Fig. 3. Non-Hodgkin diffuse large B-cell lymphoma involving a cervical lymph node, with large pleomorphic lymphoma cells (hematoxylin-eosin, original magnification ×250).

pregnancy is thought to be 0.8 cases per 100,000 women [29]. The exact prevalence of NHL during pregnancy, however, is unknown. In 1993, Hurley and coworkers [30], in a review of the current literature, reported only 103 cases of NHL occurring coincident with pregnancy or the immediate postpartum period. Since that report, however, there have been an additional 35 cases reported in association with pregnancy [31–45].

The etiology for most NHLs is not clearly defined; however, a number of well-defined risk factors have been reported. Viral agents, most notably Epstein-Bar virus, human T-cell lymphotropic virus, hepatitis C virus, and HIV, have all been associated with one or another form of NHL [29,42]. Multiple autoimmune diseases, including Sjögren's disease, lupus erythematosus, and rheumatoid arthritis, have also been implicated in the development of NHL [29,42].

Immunosuppression, whether primary or iatrogenic, is well established as a risk factor for the development of NHL [43]. This association has tempted some authors to speculate that the reported diminution in cellular immune response associated with pregnancy could adversely affect either the stage at diagnosis or the progression of these neoplasms during pregnancy [44,46]. Others, however, have suggested that the apparent association with more aggressive types of NHL and overall worse prognosis is more a result of a delay in diagnosis or a reluctance to use chemotherapy during gestation, than by pregnancy itself [16, 47,48].

Most patients (66%) present with lymphadenopathy, and only 20% of patients present with B-symptoms (night sweats, weight loss, or fever). Bone marrow involvement is found more frequently in the indolent lymphomas (39%) than with the more aggressive, high-grade, varieties (18%) [49]. Unlike high-grade lymphomas, however, the prognosis does not seem to be altered by the presence of bone marrow involvement with the more indolent types of lymphomas. Patients with T-cell lymphomas present more often with constitutional symptoms, extranodal disease, and have a poorer prognosis than those with B-cell lymphomas [50]. Burkitt's lymphoma (a B-cell NHL), however, is one of the most aggressive malignancies known and B-symptoms are often present.

The initial approach to the patient with NHL is similar to that used in patients with HL. Most patients are diagnosed based on pathologic findings of a lymph node biopsy. Importantly, however, extranodal involvement is usually widespread by the time the peripheral lymph nodes are involved. For this reason, although an accurate anatomic staging (based on the Ann Arbor staging system) is still important, staging laparotomy is not used. Furthermore, in the nonpregnant population, CT scans of the chest, abdomen, and pelvis have largely replaced lymphangiograms. During pregnancy, MRI, in addition to avoiding radiation exposure to the fetus, provides not only information regarding extranodal involvement, but possible bone marrow involvement. Both gallium and thallium scanning, although of prognostic value, are contraindicated during pregnancy.

The classification systems for the NHLs have changed numerous times over the last 40 years. The most recent system, the WHO classification, incorporates morphologic, genetic, immunophenotypic, and clinical features in organizing these malignancies [51]. In this classification scheme, NHL are divided into precursor and mature B-cell neoplasms, and precursor and mature T-cell or NK-cell neoplasms. Further refinement is based on cytogenetic studies. This system has been shown clinically to provide a higher degree of diagnostic accuracy and reproducibility than the previous system [42].

Although the stage and most common histoimmunologic types of NHL may be different in pregnancy, their clinical behavior, when properly treated, does not seem to differ significantly from nonpregnant patients. Treatment choices must be based on the stage, classification, and International Prognostic Index. Recent studies in nonpregnant patients have shown that, with aggressive NHL, standard therapy with cyclophosphamide, doxorubicin, vincristine, and prednisone results in 3-year overall survival rates (53%–62%) that are not significantly different than those with other intensive chemotherapeutic regimens (48%–56%) [50,52]. Similar long-term survival rates in pregnancies complicated by NHL and treated with multiagent chemotherapy have been reported [47].

In general, women diagnosed in the third trimester and those with early stage disease tend to have a better prognosis. Unfortunately, most pregnant women with NHL have aggressive and advanced-stage disease. Because these women have a poor prognosis, standard chemotherapy should not be delayed. Those women diagnosed in the first trimester and unwilling to accept the potential risk of fetal malformations (6%–20%), should be offered pregnancy termination [48]. After the first trimester, when the risk of fetal malformations with standard multiagent chemotherapy seems negligible, pregnancy termination is not indicated for maternal benefit. Furthermore, although second- and third-trimester exposure to multiagent chemotherapy has been associated with fetal growth restriction and myelosuppression, several recent studies have shown no significant risk of fetal toxicity [13,53].

Another potential risk to the fetus and infant whose mother has NHL is maternal-fetal transmission of malignant cells. In 2002, Walker and coworkers [54], in a review of metastatic disease of the fetus or placenta, found no cases of maternal NHL metastatic to either placenta or fetus. In 1994, however, Hurley and coworkers [30] reported a maternal case of T-cell NHL, with cytologically and immunohistologically identical T-cell lymphoma developing in the infant at 2 months of age. In 1997, Megvarian-Bedoyan and coworkers [41] described a case of anaplastic large cell lymphoma metastatic to the placenta. These same authors, on review of the literature, were able to identify three additional cases of documented placental involvement by metastatic NHL. Overall, since 1992 there have been a total of eight cases of maternal NHL metastatic to the placenta, fetus, or both [30,39–41,55]. In these cases, 62% of the mothers and 25% of the infants died, presumably from complications of disseminated NHL. It has been recommended that pathologic examination of the placenta be undertaken so that appropriate and timely consideration for neonatal follow-up and treatment can be effected [30].

As with HL, cord blood should be collected as a potential source of HLA-compatible progenitor cells, in the event that bone marrow transplant is needed.

Finally, delivery should be timed to minimize the risk of pulmonary immaturity, and the risk of neonatal myelosuppression.

## Vignette 3: leukemia

A 15-year-old Hispanic woman, $G_1P_0$ at 27 weeks' gestational age, was transported to the university hospital after presenting to a local hospital with right lower extremity pain and new-onset ecchymoses with fairly extensive petechial rash. A complete blood count showed severe anemia (hemoglobin 4.6 g/dL) with thrombocytopenia (platelets of 17,000). The patient had a normal white blood cell count, but the differential was remarkable for 35% blasts on the peripheral smear (Fig. 4). Her electrolytes were normal, as were her coagulation studies. Her serum glutamic-oxaloacetic transaminase and serum glutamic-pyruvic transaminase were in the normal range as was her lactic dehydrogenase. Her urine analysis, chest radiograph, and level 2 ultrasound were unremarkable. She was transfused with packed red blood cells and platelets before undergoing bone marrow aspiration and biopsy. The morphologic and immunophenotypic findings were consistent with pre–B-cell acute lymphoblastic leukemia (Fig. 5). Cytogenetic studies were sent and later demonstrated hyperdiploidy, with 55 chromosomes, including trisomies 2, 4, 6, 8, 10, 16, 17, 18, 21, and 22. Her initial spinal fluid showed no evidence of blasts. The patient was placed in a high-risk prognostic category based on her age.

The patient and her family were counseled extensively regarding the importance of initiating chemotherapy, despite the potential risks to her fetus from prematurity, intrauterine growth restriction, and a possible increased risk of fetal demise. She was counseled that at this gestational age, there did not seem to be an increased risk of congenital birth defects attributable to the recommended chemotherapy, and that the best data, although limited, did not demonstrate any significant long-term neurologic sequelae attributable solely to chemotherapy. After consultation between the pediatric oncology and maternal-fetal medicine

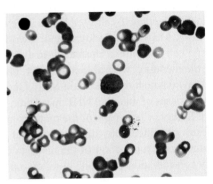

Fig. 4. Blast with lymph. Peripheral blood in pregnant woman with precursor B-cell lymphoblastic leukemia, showing lymphoblast (*center*) (Wright stain, original magnification ×1000).

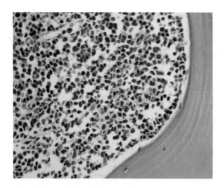

Fig. 5. Marrow core. Bone marrow biopsy in the same patient showing replacement of marrow by leukemia cells or lymphoblasts (hematoxylin-eosin, original magnification ×400).

services, the patient was offered and accepted aggressive induction chemotherapy consisting of vincristine, L-asparaginase, daunomycin, and prednisone. Methyl-prednisolone and prednisone were chosen over dexamethasone because of the concerns of repeated fetal exposure to dexamethasone and adverse neurologic sequelae. The patient also received central nervous system prophylaxis consisting of intrathecal arabinosylcytosine instead of the usual methotrexate, because of concerns for the potential toxic effect of methotrexate on trophoblastic cells. The decision was also made to maintain the patient at a hemoglobin level greater than 8 g/dL and platelet count greater than 30,000. The patient responded well to her chemotherapy and entered remission after day 8. Serial growth scans and fetal surveillance remained normal. Two weeks after initiating chemotherapy, the patient required insulin for gestational diabetes. At 31 weeks, conveniently the end of induction therapy, the patient developed symptomatic preterm labor with cervical change, and was admitted for magnesium sulfate tocolysis and antenatal corticosteroids. Her labor was successfully thwarted and she was discharged home after 4 days of observation. She developed a urinary tract infection, with methicillin-resistant enterococcus, that was successfully treated and she was placed on nitrofurantoin suppression. One day before scheduled start of consolidation chemotherapy, she developed recurrent preterm labor and it was elected to allow her labor to progress. She delivered a healthy 2086-g boy with Apgar scores of 9 and 9. The newborn showed no signs of myelosuppression and was discharged in good condition at 5 days of age. The mother's postpartum course was uneventful. She received medroxyprogesterone intramuscularly the day of delivery and was counseled against breast-feeding. She resumed her chemotherapeutic regimen 3 days postpartum.

## Leukemia

The leukemias are a heterogeneous group of malignancies that arise from genetically altered, lymphoid or myeloid progenitor cells, located in the bone marrow. This genetic abnormality results in dysregulated growth and clonal expansion. As first described by Virchow in 1845, these clonal leukemic blasts not only spill into the bloodstream, but also ultimately infiltrate liver, spleen, and other tissues [56,57]. Historically, the leukemias were classified based on their clinical presentation and life expectancy into two basic groups: acute and chronic. With advances in histochemical techniques, however, these malignancies can be further classified, based on morphologic characteristics, as being of myeloid or lymphoid cell origin: acute myeloid leukemia, chronic myeloid leukemia (CML), acute lymphoid leukemia (ALL), and chronic lymphoid leukemia (CLL). Current pathologic classification using immunophenotyping and molecular-cytogenetic studies has produced a more complex, but prognostically accurate, classification of the leukemias [58].

In the nonpregnant population, 43% of leukemias are classified as acute, whereas 41% are chronic. In pregnancy, however, most leukemias (90%) are classified as acute [25,59]. Furthermore, 68% are of myeloid cell lineage (61% acute myeloid leukemia, 7% CML), whereas 31% are of lymphoid lineage (28% ALL, 3% CLL) [60].

For most cases of leukemia, the precise causal links have not been established. There are, however, numerous associations between leukemias and various environmental, socioeconomic, infectious, and genetic events. A higher incidence of certain leukemias among monozygotic twins and syndromes with somatic cell aneuploidy (eg, Down syndrome, Patau's syndrome, and Klinefelter's syndrome) suggests a genetic etiology. Other syndromes associated with both chromosomal fragility and immune dysregulation, such as Bloom syndrome and x-linked agammaglobulinemia, also demonstrate a higher incidence of leukemia [61–64]. Numerous environmental factors, however, such as radiation exposure, exposure to alkylating agents, and certain viral infections, have been implicated in the etiology of leukemia. Known viral etiologies, including the retrovirus human T-cell lymphoma virus, are thought to play a role in adult T-cell leukemia, and Epstein-Barr virus, a DNA virus associated with mature B-cell ALL [59]. In addition, the human herpes virus-6 has been cited as a possible modulating factor in lymphocytic leukemias [65].

The clinical manifestations of the acute leukemias are nonspecific and many of these symptoms, such as fatigue, weakness, dyspnea, and lack of energy, are common in normal pregnancies. In the acute leukemias, however, they are the clinical manifestations of bone marrow infiltration by the leukemic clonal cells with resulting suppression of normal hematopoiesis. As pancytopenia progresses, however, symptoms of epistaxis, easy bruisiability, and recurrent infections should suggest a more precarious etiology. On physical examination, these patients often demonstrate pallor, petechiae, or ecchymoses. Lymphadenopathy and hepatosplenomegaly are uncommon and gingival hyperplasia, caused by leukemic cell infiltration of the gums, and cranial neuropathies may occasionally be present. In the absence of a pulmonary infection, the chest radiograph usually is normal, but may demonstrate mediastinal enlargement, particularly in patients with acute T-cell leukemia.

The diagnosis of an acute leukemia is usually suspected when a peripheral blood smear demonstrates a normocytic, normochromic anemia with a mild to severe thrombocytopenia. Although the white blood cell count is variable, blasts are virtually always present [62]. In acute promyelocytic leukemia there may be evidence of an intravascular coagulopathy, with prolongation of the partial thromboplastin time, the prothrombin time, and depression of fibrinogen, but this is a rare finding in ALL. Lumbar puncture to determine disease status in the central nervous system is recommended, and bone marrow aspiration and biopsy are essential for the diagnosis and morphologic, immunophenotypic, and cytogenetic classification of the patient's leukemia [62].

Cytogenetic abnormalities have emerged as powerful determinants of patient outcome. They are numerous in type and occur in most leukemias. The Philadelphia chromosome, translocation t (9; 22), occurs more frequently in adult ALL (25%) than in childhood ALL (3%) and is associated with a worse prognosis. The t (12; 21) translocation, seen in approximately 25% of pre–B-cell ALL, confers a favorable prognosis. Age is clearly an important prognosticator with younger patients, especially children, having a better prognosis than adults. Within the pediatric population, age continues to be a significant prognostic factor, with children diagnosed between the ages of 2 and 10 years doing better than children over 10 years at diagnosis, who in turn do better than infants. Clinically, however, the patient's rate of response to induction chemotherapy and time to normalization of bone marrow findings is one of the most useful indicators of ultimate outcome [62].

Chronic leukemias complicating pregnancy are rare, reflecting a median age of onset in the sixth decade of life. Most that do occur in pregnancy are myeloid (90%), with only four cases of CLL reported during pregnancy [66]. Only 10% of all CML cases occur during pregnancy. Chromosomal translocations, particularly the reciprocal t (9; 22)(q34; q11) and its bcr-abl fusion gene product, play a central role in the development of CML and are found in 95% of cases. The presenting symptoms of patients with CML are similar to those of acute leukemia; however, the most common sign of CML, occurring in over 90% of cases, is splenomegaly. Symptoms or signs of granulocytopenia or thrombocytopenia are uncommon and usually suggest transformation into the accelerated or blast phase. Elevated white blood cell counts, and anemia, are often seen at diagnosis. The median survival time is 4 years, with blast crisis developing 3 to 4 years after the initial diagnosis [67]. B-cell hematologic malignancies can present as either leukemia (CLL), with lymphocytosis, or as an NHL. It typically has in indolent course and may not require treatment for months to years [57].

Before the institution of modern chemotherapy, the outcome for both adults and children with acute leukemia was grim. Even today, without treatment, the average life expectancy is measured in months and not years. With treatment, however, children with ALL can now anticipate being cured of their disease 80% of the time [68]. The outcome for adults with acute leukemias, although not nearly as optimistic, has also improved with advancements in chemotherapeutic regimens and in supportive care for treatment-induced morbidities. Today, complete remission can be expected in 70% to 85% of patients, with long-term disease-free survival in 25% to 50% of patients [62].

In the patient with acute leukemia, the primary goal of chemotherapy is the eradication of leukemic clone cells from the bone marrow (less than 5% blasts) and restoration of normal hematopoiesis (granulocyte count $\geq 1000/\mu L$, platelet count $\geq 100,000/\mu L$). The secondary goal is the prevention, through the use of multiagent chemotherapeutic regimens, of the emergence of resistant clones, and through the treatment of leukemic cell sanctuaries, the elimination of residual disease. To this end, chemotherapy is divided into several phases: induction, consolidation, and maintenance [62,69].

For acute myeloid leukemia patients less than 60 years of age, remission induction typically includes the use of an anthracycline (daunorubicin or idarubicin) and cytarabine. Those who do not achieve complete remission (30% of younger adults) are candidates for allogenic hematopoietic stem cell transplant. In patients with ALL, the combination of vincristine, anthracycline, steroids, and L-asparaginase often constitutes the standard induction regimen. Newer regimens in adults with ALL, incorporating higher dose intensities, and the addition of cyclophosphamide and cytarabine have produced complete remission rates of 93%, induction mortalities of 8%, and 6-year disease-free survival of 55% [69]. Because the central nervous system is a common sanctuary for lymphocytic leukemic cells, central nervous system prophylaxis is standard therapy for adults and children with ALL. In addition to the previously mentioned chemotherapeutic drugs, patients with acute leukemia often require treatment with a pharmacopeia of other medications used in the treatment and prevention of induction-induced morbidities: allopurinol to reduce the risk of urate nephropathy; cotrimoxazole for *Pneumocystis carinii* prophylaxis; fluconazole to reduce the risk of *Candida albicans* infection; and hematopoietic growth factors (granulocyte colony–stimulating factor) to shorten the period of profound neutropenia. For most of these drugs published human experience is limited [70]. Finally, supportive measures, such as blood and platelet transfusions, and the aggressive diagnosis and treatment of febrile neutropenia, have become critical in minimizing induction morbidity and mortality [62].

The treatment of patients with chronic leukemias is individualized. For those with CLL, who present with lymphocytosis and bone marrow involvement, and for whom median survival is greater than 10 years, immediate treatment may not be required [71]. In those patients for whom treatment is deemed necessary, fludarabine is the usual treatment recommended. For those at risk of complications from thrombocytosis and leukostasis, leukapheresis may be recommended. In patients with chronic-phase CML, who are not candidates for bone marrow transplantation, imatinib is recommended as the first drug of choice [72]. In those who do not respond to imatinib, interferon-$\alpha$ has been shown to improve survival [67,71]. Leukapheresis may be used for the same indications as in CLL.

The incidence of leukemia in pregnancy is unknown, but is estimated to range from 1:75,000 to 1:100,000 pregnancies [73]. Although estrogen has been implicated in leukemic cell proliferation and estrogen receptors have been found in leukemic cell lines, it does not seem that the course of leukemia is adversely affected by pregnancy [74–77]. Unfortunately, there are no recent large reviews of pregnancy complicated by leukemia incorporating newer drug regimens and advancements in supportive care, with the largest recent series of 17 patients spanning a 37-year period [78]. Despite this, there seems to be a consensus of expert opinion that the outcome of pregnant patients with acute leukemia is adversely affected only when appropriate therapy is withheld for more than a few weeks [77–79]. Reported complete remission in pregnancies complicated by acute leukemia and aggressively treated with chemotherapy does not seem to be substantively different from those in the nonpregnant adult population [25,78,79]. Regardless of gestational age, the immediate induction of remission, as in the nonpregnant population, remains the first objective in the management of the pregnant patient with acute leukemia.

Just as in the nonpregnant patient, supportive care is also critical. Maintenance goals should include a platelet count of $\geq 30,000/\mu L$, or $\geq 50,000/\mu L$ in the presence of bleeding or at the time of delivery to allow for regional anesthesia [80]. The maternal hemoglobin should be maintained above the lower ($\pm 2$ SD) limits of 9.8 mg/dL, because the risk of perinatal complications (preterm labor, intrauterine growth restriction, and fetal demise) increase progressively as the hemoglobin declines [81].

When deciding on chemotherapeutic options, the physiologic adaptations of pregnancy need to be taken into consideration. Pregnancy is known to be a thrombogenic state, with the risk of thromboembolism six times higher than in the nonpregnant individual. L-Asparaginase, derived from either *Escherichia coli* or *Erwinia crysanthemi*, significantly decreases the levels of certain thrombosis inhibitors (eg, antithrombin III) and in children and adults with ALL has been associated with a significant risk of thromboembolism [82–85] The use of this agent in pregnancy complicated by ALL should be approached with caution. Pregnancy is also a state of increased insulin resistance. It is not surprising that the concomitant use of high doses of glucocorticoids may exacerbate what is otherwise a mild degree of carbohydrate intolerance. In addition to the effect of steroids on maternal glucose homeostasis, the type of steroid used may also be important in terms of potential adverse fetal effects. Most chemotherapeutic protocols prefer dexamethasone because of its improved central nervous system penetration. Neonatal data, however, have demonstrated a threefold increased risk of leukomalacia and neurodevelopmental abnormalities in infants exposed to repeated doses of dexamethasone for induction of fetal lung maturity [86].

The management of the chronic leukemias in pregnancy is not well defined because of the paucity of cases reported. Maternal and fetal outcomes are generally excellent, with maternal and fetal survival rates of 96% and 84%, respectively [87]. Therapy is generally aimed at controlling splenomegaly, leukocytosis, and constitutional symptoms. Interferon-α, which does not seem to cross the placental barrier to any appreciable degree, has been used in at least 10 cases of CML complicating pregnancy without adverse maternal effects, with only one case of transient neonatal thrombocytopenia [67,88]. Of the four cases of CLL complicating pregnancy, only one patient required treatment with anything other than antibiotic and blood transfusions for symptomatic anemia. She was treated with leukapheresis three times, starting in the second trimester and neither she nor her baby suffered any ill effects [66].

The effects of acute leukemia on pregnancy have not been recently studied. From the available literature, it seems that acute leukemia and or its treatment may have a detrimental effect on pregnancy outcome. Premature births occur either iatrogenically or spontaneously in over 50% of cases. Stillbirths have been reported in from 7% to 17% of cases and intrauterine growth restriction in approximately 8% of infants [17,23,25,28]. Furthermore, neonatal deaths from neutropenia and cardiomyopathy have also been reported [23,89]. The risk for adverse outcome is greatest for those diagnosed in the first trimester, but can occur in any trimester [23,77,78]. The risk of teratogenicity seems to be confined to the first 12 weeks of gestation, with folate antagonists and alkylating agents posing the greatest risk [90]. Whether methotrexate, the chemotherapeutic agent preferred for trophoblastic disease, poses a greater risk for adverse fetal outcome (excluding fetal anomalies) in the second or third trimester is neither substantiated nor refuted by the currently available literature [23,90]. What is clear from the literature, however, is that delaying appropriate chemotherapy for more than a few weeks at any time other than the latter part of the third trimester is associated with excessive fetal mortality (29%) [25,60,78].

Both NHL and leukemia metastatic to the fetus or placenta have been documented, albeit rarely. As a group, however, leukemia and lymphoma account for 19% of the malignancies metastatic to the products of conception and 50% of those metastatic to the fetus [2,54]. The placenta should always be sent for histo-pathologic evaluation. Because patients often require prolonged maintenance therapy, and because they are at significant risk of recurrence even if complete remission occurs, they should be provided with effective and reliable contraception. In addition, although the data on most of the agents used for chemotherapy and breast-feeding are scarce, patients should be instructed to avoid breast-feeding during chemotherapy.

**Summary**

Hematologic malignancies occurring during pregnancy are fortunately uncommon. When they do collide, their inherent and diametrically opposed natures, life-giving and life-threatening, create fear and anxiety for the patient, her family, and all of those who are charged with her care. It is imperative that physicians and health care providers approach these patients and their families with compassion, empathy, and most importantly the knowledge and expertise necessary to optimize the outcome for both mother and baby. Inherent conflicts between maternal and fetal well-being must be dealt with in an honest and nonjudgmental fashion. Finally, frequent communication and a spirit of teamwork between the various specialists involved in her care go far in alleviating the patient's fears and ensuring a favorable outcome.

## References

[1] Smith LH, Danielsen B, Allen ME, et al. Cancer associated with obstetric delivery: results of linkage with the California cancer registry. Am J Obstet Gynecol 2003;189:1128–35.

[2] Dildy GA, Moise KJ, Carpenter RJ, et al. Maternal malignance metastatic to the products of conception: a review. Obstet Gynecol Surv 1989;44:535–40.

[3] Pavlidis NA. Coexistence of pregnancy and malignancy. Oncologist 2002;7:279–87.

[4] Peleg D, Ben-Ami M. Lymphoma and leukemia complicating pregnancy. Obstet Gynecol Clin North Am 1998;25:365–83.

[5] Lishner M, Zemlickis D, Degendorfer P, et al. Maternal and fetal outcome following Hodgkin's disease in pregnancy. Br J Cancer 1992;65:114–7.

[6] Kadin ME. Pathology of Hodgkin's disease. Curr Opin Oncol 1994;6:456–63.

[7] Joy A, Zander T, Kornacker M. Detection of identical-Hodgkin-Reed Sternberg cell specific immunoglobulin gene rearrangements in a patient with Hodgkin's disease of mixed cellularity subtype at primary diagnosis and in relapse two and a half years later. Ann Oncol 1998;9:283–7.

[8] Longo DL, Glatstein E, Duffey PL, et al. Radiation therapy versus combination chemotherapy in the treatment of early-stage Hodgkin's disease: seven-year results of a prospective randomized trial. J Clin Oncol 1991;9:897–901.

[9] Carbone PP, Kaplan HS, Musshoff K, et al. Report of the committee on Hodgkin's disease staging classification. Cancer Res 1971;31:1860–1.

[10] Connors JM. Hodgkin's lymphoma. In: Meloni D, Morrissey D, O'Keefe K, et al, editors. Abeloff: clinical oncology. 3rd edition. Philadelphia: Elsevier; 2004. p. 2985–3014.

[11] Ward FT, Weiss RB. Lymphoma and pregnancy. Semin Oncol 1989;16:397–409.

[12] Lishner M, Zemlickis D, Degendorfer P. Maternal and fetal outcome following Hodgkin's disease in pregnancy. In: Koren G, Lishner M, Farine D, editors. Cancer in pregnancy: maternal and fetal risk. Cambridge: Cambridge University Press; 1996. p. 107–15.

[13] Aviles A, Neri N. Hematological malignancies and pregnancy: a final report of 84 children who received chemotherapy in utero. Clin Lymphoma 2001;2:173–7.

[14] Barry RM, Diamond HD, Graver LF. Influence of pregnancy on the course of Hodgkin's disease. Am J Obstet Gynecol 1962;84:445–54.

[15] Weisz B, Schiff E, Lishner M. Cancer in pregnancy: maternal and fetal implications. Hum Reprod Update 2001;7:384–93.

[16] Gelb AB, Van de Rijn M, Warnke RA, et al. Pregnancy associated lymphomas: a clinicopathologic study. Cancer 1996;78:304–10.

[17] Sweet Jr DL. Malignant lymphoma: implications during the reproductive years and pregnancy. J Reprod Med 1976;17:198–208.

[18] Vassilakopoulos TP, Angelopoulou MK, Siakantaris MP, et al. Combination chemotherapy plus low-dose involved-field radiotherapy for early clinical stage Hodgkin's lymphoma. Int J Radiat Oncol Biol Phys 2004;59:765–81.

[19] Woo SY, Fuller LM, Cundiff JH, et al. Radiotherapy during pregnancy for clinical stages IA-IIA Hodgkin's disease. Int J Radiat Oncol Biol Phys 1992;23:407–12.

[20] Brent RL. Utilization of developmental basic science principles in the evaluation of reproductive risk from pre- and postconception environmental radiation exposures. Teratology 1999;59: 182–204.

[21] Miller RW. Severe mental retardation and cancer among atomic bomb survivors exposed in utero. Teratology 1999;59:234–5.

[22] DePalma RT, Leveno KJ, Kelly MA, et al. Birth weight threshold for postponing preterm birth. Am J Obstet Gynecol 1992;167(4 Pt 1):1145–9.

[23] Cardonick E, Iacobucci A. Use of chemotherapy during human pregnancy. Lancet Oncol 2004;5: 283–91.

[24] Veradi G, Elchalal U, Shushan A. Umbilical cord blood for use in transplantation. Obstet Gynecol Surv 1995;50:611–7.

[25] Reynoso EE, Shepherd FA, Messner HA, et al. Acute leukemia during pregnancy: the Toronto Leukemia Study Group experience with long-term follow-up of children exposed in utero to chemotherapeutic agents. J Clin Oncol 1987;5:1098–106.

[26] Economopoulos T, Papageongious S, Dimopoulos MA, et al. Non-Hodgkin's lymphomas in Greece according to the WHO classification of lymphoid neoplasms: a retrospective analysis of 810 cases. Acta Haematol 2005;113:97–103.

[27] Carbone A, Franceschis S, Gloghini A, et al. Pathologic and immunophenotypic features of adult non-Hodgkin's lymphomas by age group. Hum Pathol 1997;28:580–7.

[28] Ioachim HL. Non-Hodgkin's lymphoma in pregnancy: three cases and review of the literature. Arch Pathol Lab Med 1985;109:803–9.

[29] Kuzel TM, Benson AB. Non-Hodgkin's lymphoma. In: Gleicher N, editor. Principles and practice of medical therapy in pregnancy. 2nd edition. East Norwalk (CT): Appleton and Lang; 1992. p. 1078–81.

[30] Hurley TJ, Montgomery R, Waldron J, et al. Fatal course of malignant non-Hodgkin's lymphoma of T-cell type during pregnancy with metastasis to the fetus. J Matern Fetal Med 1994;3:69–74.

[31] Stewart KS, Gordon MC. Non-Hodgkin lymphoma in pregnancy presenting as acute liver failure. The American College of Obstetricians and Gynecologists. Obstetrics Gynecology 1999; 94(S/pt2):847.

[32] Barnes MN, Barrett JC, Kimberlin DF, et al. Burkitt lymphoma in pregnancy. Obstet Gynecol 1998;92:675–8.

[33] Goldwasser F, Pico JL, Cerrina J, et al. Successful chemotherapy including epirubium in a pregnant non-Hodgkin's lymphoma patient. Leuk Lymphoma 1995;20:173–6.

[34] Spitzer M, Citron M, Llandi CF, et al. Non-Hodgkin's lymphoma during pregnancy. Gynecol Oncol 1991;43:309–12.

[35] Morice P, Cristalli B, Heid M, et al. Pregnancy and non-Hodgkin's lymphoma: a case. J Gynecol Obstet Biol Reprod (Paris) 1993;22:68–70.

[36] Lees CC, Tsirigotis M, Carr JV, et al. T-cell non-Hodgkin's lymphoma presenting in the first trimester of pregnancy. Postgrad Med J 1994;70:371–2.

[37] Silva PT, de Almeida HM, Principe F, et al. Non-Hodgkin lymphoma during pregnancy: case report. Eur J Obstet Gynecol Reprod Biol 1998;77:249–51.

[38] Aghadivno PU, Akang EEU, Ihekwuba FN, et al. Simultaneous bilateral malignant breast neoplasms in Nigerian women. J Natl Med Assoc 1994;86:365–8.

[39] Nishi Y, Suzuki S, Otsubo Y, et al. B-cell-type malignant lymphoma with placental involvement. J Obstet Gynaecol Res 2000;26:39–43.

[40] Maruko K, Maeda T, Kamitomo M, et al. Transplacental transmission of maternal B-cell lymphoma. Am J Obstet Gynecol 2004;191:380–1.

[41] Megvarian–Bedoyan Z, Lamant L, et al. Anaplastic large cell lymphoma of maternal origin involving the placenta: case report and literature survey. Am J Surg Pathol 1997;21:1236–41.

[42] Weinshel EL, Peterson BA. Hodgkin's disease. CA Cancer J Clin 1993;43:327–45.

[43] Hoover RN. Lymphoma risks in populations with altered immunity: a search for mechanisms. Cancer Res 1992;52:5477–8.

[44] Giovannini M, Saccucci P, Cannone D, et al. Can pregnancy aggravate the course of non-Hodgkin's lymphoma? Eur J Gynaecol Oncol 1989;10:287–9.

[45] Valenzuela PL, Montalban C, Matorras R, et al. Pregnancy and relapse of peripheral T-cell lymphoma. Gynecol Obstet Invest 1991;32:59–61.

[46] Selvais PL, Mazy G, Gosseye S, et al. Breast infiltration by acute lymphoblastic leukemia during pregnancy. Am J Obstet Gynecol 1993;169:1619–20.

[47] Aviles A, Diaz-Maqueo JC, Tomas V, et al. Non-Hodgkin's lymphomas and pregnancy: presentation of 16 cases. Gynecol Oncol 1990;37:335–7.

[48] Pohlman B, Macklis RM. Lymphoma and pregnancy. Semin Oncol 2000;27:657–66.

[49] Conlan MG, Bast M, Armitage JO, et al. Bone marrow involvement by non-Hodgkin's lymphoma: the clinical significance of morphologic discordance between the lymph node and bone marrow. Nebraska Lymphoma Study Group. J Clin Oncol 1990;8:1163–72.

[50] Escalon MP, Liu NS, Yang Y, et al. Prognostic functions and treatment of patients with T-cell non-Hodgkin's lymphoma. Cancer 2005;103:2091–8.

[51] Harris NL, Jaffe ES, Dicbold J, et al. World Health Organization classification of neoplastic diseases of the hematopoichic and lymphoid tissues: report of the Clinical Advisory Committee Meeting-Airlie House, Virginia, November 1997. J Clin Oncol 1999;17:3835.

[52] Lopez-Guillermo A, Garcia-Conde J, Alvarez-Carmona AM. Comparison of chemotherapy CHOP vs. CHOP/VIA in the treatment of aggressive non-Hodgkin's lymphoma: a randomized multicenter study of 132 patients. The PETHEMA Group. Med Clin (Barc) 1998;110:601–4.

[53] Cardonick E, Stepannk K, Kautmann M. The effects of chemotherapy in the midtrimester of pregnancy. Am J Obstet Gynecol 2001;185(6):S167.

[54] Walker JW, Reinisch JF, Monforte HL. Maternal pulmonary adenocarcinoma metastatic to the fetus: first recorded case report and literature review. Pediatr Pathol Mol Med 2002;21:57–69.

[55] Catin EA, Roberts JD, Erana R, et al. Transplacental transmission of natural-killer-cell lymphoma. N Engl J Med 1999;341:85–91.

[56] Yahia C, Hyman GA, Phillups LL. Acute leukemia and pregnancy. Obstet Gynecol Surv 1958;13:1–21.

[57] Armitage J, Longo D. Malignancies of lymphoid cells. In: Braunwald E, Hausser S, Fancis A, et al, editors. Harrison's: principles of internal medicine. 15th edition. New York: McGraw-Hill; 2001. p. 715–27.

[58] Kantanjiano HM, Faderl S. Acute lymphoid leukemia in adults. In: Meloni D, Mornissey D, O'Keefe K, et al, editors. Abeloff: clinical oncology. 3rd edition. Philadelphia: Elsevier; 2004. p. 2793–8.

[59] Applegaum FF. Acute myeloid leukemia in adults. In: Meloni D, Mornissey D, O'Keefe K, et al, editors. Abeloff: clinical oncology. 3rd edition. Philadelphia: Elsevier; 2004. p. 2825–42.

[60] Caligiuri MA, Mayer RJ. Pregnancy and leukemia. Semin Oncol 1989;16:338–96.

[61] McDunn SH, Winter JN. Acute leukemia. In: Gleicher N, editor. Principles and practice of medical therapy in pregnancy. 2nd edition. New York: Appleton and Lange; 1992. p. 1064–8.

[62] Hoelzer D, Gokbuget N. Acute lymphocytic leukemia in adults. In: Hoffman R, Benz EJ, Shattil SJ, editors. Hematology: basic principles and practice. 4th edition. Philadelphia: Elsevier; 2005. p. 1177.

[63] Shaw MP, Eden OB, Grace E, et al. Acute lymphoblastic leukemia and Klinefelter's syndrome. Pediatr Hematol Oncol 1992;9:81–5.

[64] Janik-Mosfant A, Bubala H, Stojewska M, et al. Acute lymphoblastic leukemia in children with Fanconi anemia. Wiad Lek 1998;51(Suppl 4):285–8.

[65] Daibata M, Taguchi T, Kemioka M, et al. Identification of integrated human herpes-virus 6 DNA in early pre-B cell acute lymphoblastic leukemia. Leukemia 1998;12:1002–5.

[66] Ali R, Ozkalemkas F, Ozkocaman V, et al. Successful labor in the course of chronic lymphocytic leukemia (CLL) and management of CLL during pregnancy with leukapheresis. Ann Hematol 2004;83:61–3.

[67] Mesquita M, Pestana A, Mota A. Successful pregnancy occurring with interferon-alpha therapy in chronic myeloid leukemia. Acta Obstet Gynecol 2005;84:300–1.

[68] Berg SL, Steuber CY, Poplack DG. Clinical manifestations of acute lymphoblastic leukemia. In: Hoffman R, Benze J, Shattil SJ, editors. Hematology: basic principles and practice. 4th edition. Philadelphia: Elsevier; 2005. p. 1155–62.

[69] Todeschini G, Tecchio C, Meneghini V, et al. Estimated 6-year event-free survival of 55% in 60 consecutive adult acute lymphoblastic leukemia patients treated with an intensive phase II protocol based on high induction dose of daunorubicin. Leukemia 1998;12:144–9.

[70] Reprotox database. Reproductive Toxicology Center, 1994–2001. Last update October 2004, cases #86386-73-4 and 62683-29-8. Available at: http://reprotox.org.

[71] Baustian GH, Fenni FF, Clark OA, et al. Chronic lymphocytic leukemia: treatment. In: Clark OA, editor. http://www.firstconsult.com First Consult Website ("site"). Oxford: Elsevier; 2005. p. 1 (Part 4).

[72] Kabonjo M, O'Handon KM, Clark OA, et al. Chronic myelogenous leukemia: summary. In: Clark OA, editor. http://www.firstconsult.com First Consult Website ("site"). Oxford: Elsevier; 2005. p. 1 (Part 4).

[73] Bartsch HH, Meyer D, Teichmann AT, et al. Treatment of promyelocytic leukemia during pregnancy. Blat 1988;57:51–4.

[74] Bishop JM. Oncogenes as hormone receptors. Nature 1986;321:112–3.

[75] Caligiuni MA, Mayer RJ. Pregnancy and leukemia. Semin Oncol 1989;16:388–96.

[76] Daniel L, Condien B, Revillard JP, et al. Presence of oestrogen binding sites and growth-stimulating effect of oestradiol in human myelogenous cell line HL 60. Cancer 1986;42:4701–5.

[77] Catanzanite VA, Ferguson JE. Acute leukemia and pregnancy: a review of management and outcome. Obstet Gynecol Surv 1984;39:663–78.

[78] Greenlund LJS, Letendne L, Tefferi A. Acute leukemia during pregnancy: a single institutional experience with 17 cases. Leuk Lymphoma 2001;41:571–7.

[79] Kaloamura S, Yoshiike M, Shimoyama T, et al. Management of acute leukemia during pregnancy: from the results of a nation wide questionnaire survey and literature survey. Tohoku J Exp Med 1944;174:167–75.

[80] McCrae KR, Russel JB, Mannucci PM, et al. Platelets: an update on diagnosis and management of thrombocytopenic disorders. Hematology (Am Soc Hematol Educ Program) 2001;1:282–305.

[81] Sifakis S, Pharmakides G. Anemia in pregnancy. Ann N Y Acad Sci 2000;900:125–36.

[82] Elliott MA, Wolf RC, Hook CC, et al. Thromboembolism in adults with acute lymphoblastic leukemia during induction with L-asparaginase-containing multi-agent regimens: incidence, risk factors, and possible role of antithrombin. Leuk Lymphoma 2004;45:1545–51.

[83] Beinant G, Damon L. Thrombosis associated with L-asparaginase therapy and low fibrinogen levels in adult acute lymphoblastic leukemia. Am J Hematol 2004;77:331–5.

[84] Mauz-Konholz C, Junken R, Gobel U, et al. Prothrombotic risk factors in children with acute lymphoblastic leukemia treated with delayed E. coli asparaginase CCOALL-92 and 97 protocols. Thromb Haemost 2000;83:840–3.

[85] Jaime-Perez JC, Gomez-almaguer D. The complex nature of the prothrombotic state in acute lymphoblastic leukemia of childhood. Haematology 2003;88:ELT25.

[86] Syinillo A, Viazzo F, Colleoni R, et al. Two-year infant neurodevelopmental outcome after single or multiple antenatal courses of corticosteroids to prevent complications of prematurity. Am J Obstet Gynecol 2004;191:217–24.

[87] Sadural E, Smith LG. Hematologic malignancies during pregnancy. Clin Obstet Gynecol 1995;38:525–46.

[88] Mutarak AA, Kakil ER, Awidi A, et al. Normal outcome of pregnancy in chronic myeloid leucemia treated with interferon-alpha in 1st trimester: report of 3 cases and review of the literature. Am J Hematol 2002;69:115–8.

[89] Achtani C, Hohlfeld P. Cardiotoxic transplacental effect of idarubicin administered during the second trimester of pregnancy. Am J Obstet Gynecol 2000;183:511–2.

[90] Leslie KK. Chemotherapy and pregnancy. Clin Obstet Gynecol 2002;5:153–64.

ELSEVIER
SAUNDERS

Obstet Gynecol Clin N Am
32 (2005) 615–626

OBSTETRICS AND
GYNECOLOGY
CLINICS
OF NORTH AMERICA

# Gestation Trophoblastic Diseases: Management of Cases with Persistent Low Human Chorionic Gonadotropin Results

Laurence A. Cole, PhD[a],*, Ernest Kohorn, MD[b],
Harriet O. Smith, MD[c]

[a]*Division of Women's Health Research, Department of Obstetrics and Gynecology,
University of New Mexico Health Sciences Center, 2211 Lomas Boulevard, NE,
Albuquerque, NM 87131–5286, USA*
[b]*Department of Obstetrics and Gynecology, Yale University School of Medicine, FMB 332,
333 Cedar Street, New Haven, CT 06510, USA*
[c]*Division of Gynecologic Oncology, Department of Obstetrics and Gynecology,
University of New Mexico Health Sciences Center, 2211 Lomas Boulevard, NE,
Albuquerque, NM 87131–5286, USA*

In the months following evacuation of a hydatidiform mole or chemotherapy treatment for persistent mole, gestational trophoblastic malignancy ([GTM], a generic term for a trophoblastic malignancy without histology) or choriocarcinoma, it is not uncommon for patients to develop persistent low human chorionic gonadotropin (hCG) results. Specifically, these are hCG values that have diminished and plateaued, and are persistent, not rising, hCG results. Alternatively, following a variable period with undetectable hCG results, a few patients under surveillance are found to have serum hCG titers that slowly rise and then plateau, and persist, with minimally fluctuating hCG results [1–7]. There are also many cases in which persistent low hCG results are detected in the months after treatment of an ectopic pregnancy, after a spontaneous miscarriage, or following a term pregnancy [1–5]. Finally, there are cases of low hCG values that persist in asymptomatic women, with or without history of gestational trophoblastic disease, which are discovered by an incidental serum pregnancy test before an elective surgical procedure, or at the time of a scheduled hCG test [1–5,8–18].

* Corresponding author.
*E-mail address:* lcole@salud.unm.edu (L.A. Cole).

*obgyn.theclinics.com*

Adding to the confusion, women in perimenopause, postmenopause, or post-oophorectomy occasionally can also have persistent low levels of hCG that is not associated with gestational trophoblastic disease or pregnancy, and seems to be a normal finding [1,3,7,19–22]. All of these situations meet the criteria for persistent low hCG result syndromes.

The finding of persistent low levels of hCG raises concern, regardless of the antecedent history, and often provokes the evaluating physician to embark on further work-up. When dilation and curettage, laparoscopy, or radiographic evaluation (ultrasound, CT scan, chest radiograph) reveal no intrauterine pregnancy or evidence of GTM or choriocarcinoma, a patient is likely to be referred to a medical or gynecologic oncologist for further evaluation and treatment, and until recently it was not uncommon for these patients to undergo chemotherapy or hysterectomy for presumed GTM, placental site trophoblastic disease, or choriocarcinoma. In patients who have a positive hCG result, any CT or MRI irregularity is likely to be considered a tumor. When the chemotherapy or hysterectomy fails to suppress the hCG production, even more invasive therapy or additional cytotoxic chemotherapy may be given.

The USA hCG Reference Service was started in 1998 to aid physicians with these persistent low hCG cases (www.hcglab.com). A serum and urine sample is submitted for a consultation with the service along with all pertinent patient records. Multiple hCG and hCG-related molecule tests are run to investigate the source and nature of the hCG to determine if the hCG is real or a mimicking molecule, and to determine if it is actually coming from trophoblast cells. Specific assays are able to determine if the value is derived from invasive or malignant cells. A formal report is prepared along with recommendations. This article reviews the observations of the USA hCG Reference Service for 134 cases with persistent low hCG results. Examination of these cases provides clear insight for the appropriate management of those presenting with persistent low levels of hCG. Although well intentioned, as these collective medial reports reveal, some women underwent hysterectomy and even more invasive surgeries, and in many cases multiple cycles of chemotherapy that was not only unnecessary but in some cases harmful. Tragically, at least one patient died from such therapy. The goal from discussion of these 134 cases is to inform practicing obstetricians and gynecologists of the reality of quiescent hCG, phantom hCG in suspected GTM cases, and normal hCG in patients who historically were thought not to manifest hCG (perimenopausal women, women on oral contraceptives who are not pregnant and who do not have gestational trophoblastic neoplasia) and to avoid unnecessary therapy.

Three distinct sources are discussed for persistent low hCG results: (1) quiescence gestational trophoblastic disease; (2) false-positive hCG results; and (3) pituitary hCG. For all three of these conditions, neither chemotherapy nor hysterectomy is likely to suppress hCG production [1–22]. Before starting chemotherapy or surgery, even if the patient has a recent history of hydatidiform mole or hCG-producing malignant disease, it is necessary to consider these three potential sources of hCG in cases that have persistent low levels of hCG.

On receipt of medical reports and serum and urine samples (a referral) the USA hCG Reference Service first excludes false-positive hCG. Three criteria are used to identify false-positive hCG results:

1. The presence of hCG immunoreactivity in serum but not urine. Heterophilic antibodies or human antianimal immunoglobulin is the cause of most false-positive serum hCG results. These rarely cross the glomerular basement membrane and enter urine. A urine pregnancy test is negative in these cases.
2. Variable hCG results (more than fivefold) or negative results in any of three or more hCG tests (caused by variable reaction with heterophilic antibodies).
3. The suppression of positive hCG result by a heterophilic antibody blocking agent (Scantibodies, San Diego, CA). If the hCG is real, then an invasive or noninvasive trophoblast, nontrophoblastic neoplasm, or hCG of pituitary origin is considered. Hyperglycosylated hCG (Hg-hCG) is a carbohydrate variant of hCG made only by trophoblast stem cells, or cytotrophoblast cells [23,24]. Hg-hCG is the principal component of hCG in very early pregnancy, at the time of implantation, and in active choriocarcinoma or GTM [1,3,24–26], conditions marked by cytotrophoblast cells. It is a marker of invasive trophoblast cells [1,3,25,26]. The USA hCG Reference Service uses the Food and Drug Administration approved automated Hg-hCG test, Advantage ITA (Nichols Institute Diagnostics, San Clemente, CA), and automated total hCG test, Immulite hCG (DPC, Los Angeles, CA), to measure the two markers and to calculate the proportion of hCG immunoreactivity caused by Hg-hCG. In the experience of the USA hCG Reference Service, the proportion Hg-hCG is 50% ± 39% in 79 cases with choriocarcinoma or GTM and advancing hCG results, compared with 9.4% ± 7.2% in 55 cases with advancing hydatidiform mole. No overlap was observed in these two groups, indicating 100% detection of invasive disease at 0% false-positive [1–5,7]. Similarly, measurement of the proportion Hg-hCG clearly distinguishes early (N = 46, 25% ± 13%) and advanced (N = 33, 83% ± 39%) choriocarcinoma or GTM ($P = .000001$). The USA hCG Reference Service measures the proportion of Hg-hCG. It uses this assay, along with persistence of hCG results or rising hCG results, to differentiate active (requires intervention for GTM) and most probably inactive gestational trophoblastic disease [1–5].

Germ cell and nontrophoblastic neoplasms characteristically produce the free β-subunit of hCG [27–31]. The free β-subunit is degraded into β-core fragment, the terminal degradation product in urine. The Service uses free β-subunit measurements (DPC Immulite free β-subunit test) and β-core fragment measurements (in-house immunometric assay) to identify these molecules. The authors have also found that free β-subunit is also the primary immunoreactivity in cases of placental site trophoblastic tumor, permitting discrimination of this from other forms of gestational trophoblastic disease [32]. In women older that 45 years, the pituitary can account for up to 25 mIU/mL hCG [20,33]. Pituitary hCG (suppressed by therapy with estrogen-progesterone combination) may be considered in these cases.

Table 1
The US hCG Reference Service experience with 134 cases with persistent low levels of hCG with no evidence of pregnancy or imaging evidence of tumor

| | |
|---|---|
| *Quiescent GTD* | |
| History of cases | |
| History of hydatidiform mole | 35 |
| History of GTM or choriocarcinoma | 6 |
| History of ectopic, aborted, or term pregnancy | 11 |
| Total cases | 52 |
| Cases receiving needless therapy (%) | 35 (67) |
| hCG and related test results | |
| hCG level at time of referral (mean ± SD) | 31 ± 32 mIU/mL |
| Range of hCG levels at time of referral | 0.5–144 mIU/mL |
| Range of hCG results until referral | <2 to 773 mIU/mL |
| Duration of persistent results before referral | 3 month to 16 years |
| Proportion of Hg-hCG at referral | 50 cases, Hg-hCG undetectable |
| | 1 case 10% and 1 12% with histories of |
| | >6 months nonrising hCG levels |
| Outcome after referral (50% reporting) | |
| Cases in which choriocarcinoma or GTM develops | 11 |
| Cases dissipating within 6 months of referral | 18 |
| | |
| *False-positive HCG* | |
| History of cases | |
| History of hydatidiform mole | 9 |
| History of GTM or choriocarcinoma | 3 |
| No history | 57 |
| Total cases | 69 |
| Cases receiving needless therapy (%) | 54 (78) |
| False-positive hCG results | |
| False-positive hCG result immediately before referral | 104 ± 153 IU/mL |
| Range of hCG results immediately before referral | 6.1–900 mIU/mL |
| Range of false-positive hCG at times before referral | 2–1007 mIU/mL |
| | |
| *Pituitary HCG* | |
| History of cases | |
| History of hydatidiform mole | 5 |
| History of GTM or choriocarcinoma | 1 |
| No history | 7 |
| Total cases | 13 |
| Cases receiving needless therapy (%) | 2 (15) |
| hCG test results | |
| hCG level at time of referral (mean ± SD) | 8.2 ± 5.2 mIU/mL |
| Range of hCG levels at time of referral | 1.2–19 mIU/mL |
| Range of hCG results until referral | 0.5–19 mIU/mL |

## False-positive human chorionic gonadotropin

As described in Table 1, the authors have identified using the method described previously, and confirmed (showing other tests are false-positive with blood sample or lack of hCG parallelism with dilution), false-positive hCG in 69 women. Although most cases followed no history of gestational trophoblastic disease, 12 were being monitored for hydatidiform mole, GTM, or choriocarcinoma. In this instance, finding a positive hCG test after normalization, or a plateau in the hCG titer, led to a work-up for GTM and chemotherapy was begun. Because this pattern is particularly confusing, it is imperative to exclude false-positive hCG before starting chemotherapy. This can be done by requesting that one's laboratory send the serum to an outside laboratory running an alternative hCG test. If both results are similar, then the hCG elevation is likely real hCG. Alternatively, if the serum hCG is >100 mIU/mL, a simple urine test can be used to examine the reality of the hCG. Urine tests normally have a sensitivity of 25 mIU/mL; if the urine test is positive, it is likely real hCG.

In most cases, false-positive hCG was discovered at the time of an incidental serum pregnancy test; as part of a check-up; before minor surgery; or before commencement of medication, radiograph, or other diagnostic procedures. Persistent low hCG results in the range 100 to 1000 mIU/mL over 2 to 6 weeks may be confused with an ectopic pregnancy and lead to methotrexate therapy or surgical intervention, including salpingectomy. When the hCG titer then fails to abate despite treatment, or when ectopic pregnancy has been excluded, then the diagnosis of GTM is entertained, and the patient is likely to be referred to a medical or gynecologic oncologist for intervention. The interfering agent that causes false-positive hCG results, a human antianimal immunoglobulin or human heterophilic antibody, arises from the immune system. Normally, the chemotherapy suppresses the immune system, which suppresses the interfering substance, and false hCG results decline. In the past, this apparent response to treatment was interpreted as indicative of response by real GTM or choriocarcinoma, despite the absence of visible disease on examination, chest radiograph, MRI, or CT scans. Unfortunately, once the immune system repairs itself, the false-positive hCG result returned, and more extreme therapies were commonly considered under the mistaken belief that

---

Note(s) to Table 1:

The 69 cases diagnosed as having false-positive hCG were based on multiple observations by the US hCG Reference Service. These are: (1) the presence of hCG immunoreactivity in serum but not urine; (2) varying hCG results (more than fivefold) or negative results in three or more hCG tests; and (3) the suppression of result by a heterophilic antibody blocking agent. The 13 pituitary hCG cases were defined as those with low levels of hCG (< 25 mIU/mL), in which the hCG immunoreactivity was totally suppressed after treatment with an oral progesterone-estrogen combination. In all these cases women were perimenopausal or postmenopausal. After excluding false-positive, and in pertinent cases, pituitary hCG, 52 cases were identified with low levels of hCG persisting for 3 months or longer, with no consistent incline or decline in hCG result.

*Abbreviations:* GTD, gestational trophoblastic disease; GTM, gestational trophoblastic malignancy; hCG, human chorionic gonadotropin.

the patient in fact had chemotherapy-resistant GTM. In the recent past, this led to some patients receiving multiple forms of chemotherapy and even hysterectomy for what is now understood to be a nonexistent disease. As indicated in Table 1, 54 (78%) of 69 such cases that were identified as having false-positive hCG by the Reference Service received needless therapy, ranging from single-agent methotrexate chemotherapy to multiple combinations of different chemotherapy protocols, or hysterectomy, and other surgeries.

In the authors' experience, at time of referral, the false-positive hCG value has averaged 104 ± 153 IU/mL, and has ranged from 6.1 to 900 mIU/mL. Considering all of their cases, false-positive hCG values obtained before referral have ranged from 2 to 1007 mIU/mL. Interestingly, a disproportionate number of cases have involved one manufacturer's hCG test, the Abbott AxSym total hCG test (Abbott Diagnostics, Chicago, Illinois). False-positive results in this test were responsible for 51 (74%) of the 69 cases, and almost all cases described recently by others [13–18]. A second test, the Bayer Centaur total hCG (Bayer Diagnostics, Tarrytown, New Jersey), was responsible for nine other cases (13%), whereas six other tests were responsible for one to three other false-positive tests. These data indicate that the treating physician needs to be aware of the assay being used by the center's laboratory, and if the laboratory is using the Abbott AxSym or Bayer Centaur test, an assay using an alternative system is critical before initiating further work-up or treatment. According to reports from the American College of Pathologists, the Abbott AxSym currently accounts for < 25% of hCG tests in the United States, based on the USA hCG Reference Service experiences' accounts for most false-positive tests, and almost all cases described recently by others [13–18]. The authors are informed by users that this test may account for more than half of the hCG testing performed in Mexico; the United Kingdom; Germany; and other European, Asian, and Central and South American locations. These are places where false-positive results and needless therapy will likely go ignored.

Although the exact extent of false-positive hCG results cannot be estimated, it is clearly quite common, and may be spread worldwide. In a case example, a 29-year-old woman, para 0, gravida 0, had an incidental hCG test very shortly after being married. The result was in the 600 mIU/mL range. After a pregnancy was excluded and an ectopic pregnancy unsuccessfully treated, GTM was inferred. She received methotrexate, which simply suppressed her immune system, then actinomycin D, which deceivingly did the same. At this time the hCG test results (Abbott AxSym) were questioned and serum sent to multiple other laboratories. Unfortunately, at that time the other laboratories were using the same Abbott AxSym tests, which were interpreted as confirmatory, and a hysterectomy was performed. Even this did not abate the hCG result, and she was placed on cytotoxic etoposide, methotrexate and actinomycin D, alternating with cyclophosphamide and vincristine (EMA-CO) combination chemotherapy. When the hCG continued to be in the range of 600 mIU/mL, a CT of the chest was performed and suggested a tumor-like mass. Under the belief that the site of persistent GTM had been identified, a thoracotomy was performed, but no tumor was found at pathology. The center's laboratory then contacted other outside laboratories where other assays were used, that demonstrated grossly variable results. The authors were consulted at this time, and the diagnosis of false-positive hCG was firmly demonstrated.

## Quiescent gestational trophoblastic disease

Quiescent gestational trophoblastic disease is a benign or inactive form of GTM or choriocarcinoma, marked by persistent low hCG results, relenting for periods ranging from 3 months to 16 years [1–7]. It may also be considered as a premalignant state in that a significant proportion of cases transform into GTM or choriocarcinoma [1–7]. The authors have reviewed the histology slides from two cases undergoing surgery for this condition. In both cases, intermediate and highly differentiated syncytiotrophoblast cells were observed, with a clear absence of cytotrophoblast cells that mark most cases of choriocarcinoma [1,2]. Differentiated syncytiotrophoblast cells can be slow-growing cells, rather than invasive cells. It is inferred that syncytiotrophoblast cells with the absence of cytotrophoblast cells is the nature of quiescent gestational trophoblastic disease: syncytiotrophoblast cells remaining after treatment of an ectopic pregnancy, parturition, or abortion, or following evacuation of a hydatidiform mole. Alternatively, slow-growing syncytiotrophoblast cells can remain after chemotherapeutic resolution of cytotrophoblast or following treatment of GTM or choriocarcinoma, where these cells may persist.

The USA hCG Reference Service has consulted on 57 cases with persistent low real hCG results. In all cases the persistent low levels persisted for 3 months or greater with minimal fluctuation and no clear upward or downward hCG trend. Hg-hCG was measured as a proportion of total hCG as a marker for invasive cytotrophoblast cells. Five case had highly positive Hg-hCG (>15%). In all five cases, hCG results sharply increased close to the time of referral and GTM or choriocarcinoma was diagnosed. The authors have interpreted these findings to mean that the trophoblastic cells have undergone malignant transformation. In 50 of the remaining 52 cases, which the authors class as quiescent gestation trophoblastic disease [1–7], no Hg-hCG was detected. In the other two remaining cases, 10% and 12% Hg-hCG was detected. In both, detectable hCG persisted for greater that 6 months with minimal fluctuation. Considering these histories, and that in these exceptional cases the proportion of Hg-hCG was below those of all 79 GTM or choriocarcinoma cases referred to the Service, the diagnosis of quiescent gestational trophoblastic disease was conferred. These data confirm the use of Hg-hCG as a marker for differentiating quiescent and invasive disease. Considering that Hg-hCG is only produced by cytotrophoblast cells [23,24], the absence of Hg-hCG in quiescent gestational trophoblast disease confirms its nature as syncytiotrophoblast in the absence of cytotrophoblast cells.

Of the 52 identified cases, 35 followed evacuation of a hydatidiform mole; 6 followed successful treatment of GTM or choriocarcinoma; and 11 following a spontaneously aborted, ectopic, or term pregnancy. The authors examined the medical records of the 52 identified quiescent gestational trophoblastic disease cases. Although 35 (67%) had received chemotherapy, combination chemotherapy, hysterectomy, or other surgery for assumed active disease, none fully responded to the therapy, including chemotherapy. The authors have interpreted this to mean that there are slowly growing syncytiotrophoblastic cells producing hCG. In all treated cases, hysterectomy partially but never completely suppressed the hCG result. The authors have interpreted this to mean that syncytiotrophoblast cells commonly remain outside of the uterus after a gestational event, or alternatively are transposed through the fallopian isthmus by an endometriosis-like mechanism. With a 100% summary of records indicating that therapy does not work, and similar findings by others [6,7], it is inferred that treating physicians should refrain from using chemotherapy or surgery in these cases. The authors' history with quiescent gestational trophoblastic disease cases is like that with false-positive hCG cases: too many people receiving needless therapy for a poorly understood and only recently fully recognized condition that requires no therapy. In one case, a patient was shown by the Service on two separate occasions during the course of 1 year to have quiescent disease. Despite this and the authors' recommendations, additional combinations of chemotherapeutic agents were given. This patient is now deceased; tragically, she died from complications of pulmonary fibrosis following bleomycin chemotherapy. Nevertheless, this case is important because it emphasizes the importance of making an accurate diagnosis of GTM before initiating cytotoxic chemotherapy. This requires all medical and gynecologic oncologists, and whoever manages patients who undergo hCG determinations, to be able to recognize and diagnose the phenomenon of quiescent gestational trophoblastic disease. If the diagnosis is in doubt or suspect, these data indicate the importance referring such patients to centers with experience with this condition before therapy is initiated. Among the 52 cases, persistent hCG levels at the time of referral were $31 \pm 32$ mIU/mL (see Table 1). The range of referred cases was 0.5 to 144 mIU/mL. Among patients, the extremes of quiescent disease hCG results were $< 2$ to 773 mIU/mL. The duration of quiescent gestational trophoblastic disease ranged from 3 months to 16 years (see Table 1).

The USA hCG Reference Service always requests follow-up reports on quiescent gestational trophoblastic disease cases, and to encourage follow-up, does not charge for repeat referrals on the same patient. Even so, it is estimated that only approximately half of the referring physicians send follow-up reports. For instance, the authors are aware that 18 cases self-resolved within 6 months of referral. Considering the 50% reporting estimate, it is presumed that this indicates that about 36 cases (69%) underwent spontaneous resolution. The authors were also informed that 11 (21%) cases later developed GTM or choriocarcinoma. If this is representative of half of the referrals, this means that up to 42% of these patients eventually developed a malignancy. It is the authors' experience that physicians are more inclined to follow-up with a negative or problem outcome, with a more pressing need for repeat testing, than for a self-resolving outcome.

As such, the authors conclude that the incidence of later transformation of malignancy is somewhere between 21% and 42%. The higher transformation rate is supported by the findings of others [6,7]. Considering the pure syncytiotrophoblast origin of quiescent gestational trophoblastic disease, the authors speculate that the high incidence of transformation occurs because these cells undergo apoptosis and are replaced by a transit cytotrophoblast cell stage. It is assumed that this is a rapid transformation because of the absence of Hg-hCG, and transformation from a slowly growing noninvasive cell type to malignant or GTM occurs during this transient cytotrophoblast cell stage.

Considering a probable 21% to 42% incidence of eventual trophoblastic transformation, it is essential to monitor cases very frequently with serial hCG measurements using both an hCG test and the commercial Hg-hCG test (Nichols Advantage, Invasive Trophoblast Antigen test). In the authors' experience most transformations occur within 2 years. They suggest testing cases weekly for 6 months, biweekly for 2 years, and monthly thereafter. Data indicate that therapy should be withheld until either continuously rising hCG results are observed or the hCG result exceeds the range of values observed for quiescent or inactive disease (150 mIU/mL), or when positive Hg-hCG results are observed.

A representative case is presented. A 23-year-old patient, para 0, gravida 1, had 5 months of negative hCG results following evacuation of a complete hydatidiform mole. A positive hCG was detected as part of the follow-up at 30 mIU/mL. Twenty days later no significant increase was observed (32 mIU/mL). Ultrasound of the pelvis and MRI of the brain and pelvis and CT of the abdomen revealed no abnormalities. Two courses of methotrexate were initiated for assumed scattered persistent mole. No diminution in hCG was observed (31 mIU/mL). Actinomycin D chemotherapy was then given, without diminution of hCG (34 mIU/mL). At this time dilation and curettage were performed, again revealing no trophoblastic tumor. The hCG test was repeated using another laboratory and a different test, but results were very similar. One month later, with no changes in hCG levels, the patient was referred to the USA hCG Reference Service. With the finding of the absence of Hg-hCG in serum and urine samples quiescent gestational trophoblast disease was proposed and further therapy was halted. Up until this time persistent hCG results had been recorded for 4 months, with as much as 40% fluctuation (low 15 mIU/mL, high 34 mIU/mL, median 25 mIU/mL). Three months later hCG results increased significantly, first to 79 mIU/mL and 7 days later, to 320 mIU/mL. On follow-up consultation, 37% of the hCG was now shown to be of Hg-hCG origin. Active disease was suspected, and 1 month later following hysterectomy, the diagnosis of choriocarcinoma was histologically confirmed.

**Pituitary human chorionic gonadotropin**

Gonadotrope cells of the pituitary produce luteinizing hormone and follicle-stimulating hormone during the menstrual cycle. During this time, production is stimulated by hypothalamic gonadotropin-releasing hormone, and modulated by feedback to the hypothalamus by ovarian granulosa cell estrogen and corpus luteal cell progesterone. With the approach of menopause (perimenopause) and in menopause, the diminished estrogen and progesterone production leaves gonadotropin-releasing hormone uncontrolled. The uncontrolled gonadotropin-releasing hormone stimulation classically leads to elevations in luteinizing hormone and follicle-stimulating hormone production. The hCG α-subunit is the same as luteinizing hormone and follicle-stimulating hormone α-subunit. The single luteinizing hormone β-subunit gene is buried within a sequence of seven hCG β-subunit genes. As such, it is not surprising that the perimenopausal and postmenopausal uncontrolled gonadotropin-releasing hormone stimulation can lead to hCG production by gonadotrope cells. The authors have been consulted on 13 such cases, and in all the source (hypothalamic-pituitary axis) was confirmed by showing that 2 or 3 weeks of therapy with an estrogen-progesterone combination pill completely suppressed the hCG production. In 6 of the 13 cases, there was a history of hydatidiform mole or choriocarcinoma, which led to the concern that these patients had GTM. In all 13 cases, the patients were referred with the presumptive diagnosis of malignant disease, and in two chemotherapy was initiated. In the authors' experience, the serum levels of hCG at the time of referral were 8.2 ± 5.2 mIU/mL, with a range of 1.2 to 19 mIU/mL.

## Summary

As indicated by the USA hCG Reference Service experience, despite announcements by the American College of Obstetricians and Gynecologists and the Society of Gynecologic Oncologists regarding the importance of verifying the diagnosis of GTM before initiating therapy, there continues to be confusion among clinicians who manage these patients, and unfortunately patients are continuing to receive unnecessary therapy. It is known that at least one person died as a consequence of therapy for the misdiagnosis of choriocarcinoma and GTM. The goal is to improve public awareness about conditions that mimic GTM. These include false-positive hCG, quiescent gestational trophoblastic disease, and pituitary hCG. Some of these conditions are harmless, but in the case of quiescent hCG, there is a very real possibility for malignant transformation. In this special circumstance, close follow-up is critical, but therapy should be withheld until there are sharply increasing hCG results, most notably those over 100 mIU/mL [34,35]. This is particularly relevant for the patient with a recent or remote history of hydatidiform mole or GTM. Under these circumstances, the first step is to confirm the diagnosis using a different laboratory and hCG test. If results are very different (more than twofold) then false-positive hCG is likely. If the patient is over 45 years old or postoophorectomy, then pituitary hCG should be considered as the likely cause, regardless of history, and can be confirmed with 2 weeks or so of combination estrogen-progesterone therapy, which suppresses the hCG result in patients with this diagnosis. This is in keeping with currently recommended guidelines in patients undergoing postmolar surveillance, that all such patients undergo oral contraception for up to a year following evacuation of a molar pregnancy. This practice also excludes the complications of pituitary hCG.

In patients following the diagnosis of hydatidiform mole, GTM, or choriocarcinoma, if there is complete resolution of measurable hCG, and then titers slowly rise and then plateau, this is indicative of quiescent gestational trophoblastic disease. This condition is not likely to respond to chemotherapy [1–7]. It is important to discriminate whether newly rising hCG is leading to a plateau (quiescent disease) or will continuously rise (malignant disease). In some cases, following treatment of a molar pregnancy or GTM, the hCG plateaus below 250 mIU/mL. This can also be consistent with the diagnosis of quiescent gestational trophoblastic disease, and does not respond to therapy [1–7]. The diagnosis of quiescent disease can be readily confirmed by showing the absence of Hg-hCG (< 0.3 ng/mL). This test is approved by the Food and Drug Administration and readily available at national clinical laboratories (Nichols Institute Laboratories, Invasive Trophoblast Antigen test).

## References

[1] Cole LA, Khanlian SA. Inappropriate management of women with persistent low hCG results. J Reprod Med 2004;49:423–32.
[2] Khanlian SA, Smith HO, Cole LA. Persistent low levels of hCG: a pre-malignant gestational trophoblastic disease. Am J Obstet Gynecol 2003;188:1254–9.
[3] Cole LA, Sutton JM. hCG tests in the management of gestational trophoblastic diseases. Clin Obstet Gynecol 2003;46:533–40.
[4] Cole LA. Use of hCG tests for evaluating trophoblastic diseases: choosing an appropriate hCG assay, false detection of hCG, unexplained elevated hCG, and quiescent trophoblastic disease. In: Hancock BW, Newlands ES, Berkowitz RS, et al, editors. Gestational trophoblastic disease. 2nd edition. Sheffield: Sheffield University Press; 2003. p. 130–55. Available at: http://www.isstd.org/gtd/index.html.
[5] Cole LA, Sutton JM. Selecting an appropriate hCG test for management of gestational trophoblastic diseases and cancer cases. J Reprod Med 2004;49:545–53.
[6] Hancock BW, Tidy JA. Clinical management of persistent low level hCG elevation. Trophobl Dis Upd 2004;4:5–6.
[7] Kohorn EI. Persistent low-level "real" human chorionic gonadotropin: a clinical challenge and a therapeutic dilemma. Gynecol Oncol 2002;85:315–20.
[8] Rotmensch S, Cole LA. False diagnosis and needles therapy of presumed malignant disease in women with false-positive human chorionic gonadotropin concentrations. Lancet 2000;355: 712–5.
[9] Cole LA, Butler SA. False positive or phantom hCG result: a serious problem. Clin Lab Intl 2001;25:9–14.
[10] Cole LA. Phantom hCG and phantom choriocarcinoma. Gynecol Oncol 1998;71:325–9.
[11] Cole LA, Rinne KM, Shababi S, et al. False positive hCG assay results leading to unnecessary surgery and chemotherapy and needless occurrences of diabetes and coma. Clin Chem 1999; 45:313–4.
[12] Butler SA, Cole LA. The use of heterophilic antibody blocking agent (HBT) in reducing false positive hCG results. Clin Chem 2001;47:1332–3.
[13] Vladutiu AO, Sulewski JM, Pudlak KA, et al. Heterophilic antibodies interfering with radioimmunoassay: a false-positive pregnancy test. JAMA 1982;248:2489–90.

[14] Olsen TG, Hubert PR, Nycum LR. Falsely elevated human chorionic gonadotropin leading to unnecessary therapy. Obstet Gynecol 2001;98:843–5.

[15] Chu JW, Goldman JO. False elevation of serum hCG: laboratory updates, Detroit Medical Center University Laboratories, 2003. Available at: http://www.dmc.org/univlab/jau_janice.htm.

[16] Rode L, Daugaard G, Fenger M, et al. Serum-hCG: still a problematic marker. Acta Obstet Gynecol Scand 2003;82:199–200.

[17] Esfandiari N, Goldberg JM. Heterophile antibody blocking agent to confirm false positive serum human chorionic gonadotropin assay. Obstet Gynecol 2003;101:1144–6.

[18] Billieux MH, Petignat P, Anguenot JL, et al. Early and late half-life of human chorionic gonadotropin as a predictor of persistent trophoblast after laparoscopic conservative surgery for tubal pregnancy. Acta Obstet Gynecol Scand 2003;82:550–5.

[19] Hoermann R, Spoettl G, Moncayo R, et al. Evidence for the presence of human chorionic gonadotropin (hCG) and free beta-subunit of hCG in the human pituitary. J Clin Endocrinol Metab 1990;71:179–86.

[20] Suginami H, Kawaoi A. Immunohistochemical localization of a human chorionic gonadotropin-like substance in the human pituitary gland. J Clin Endocrinol Metab 1982;55:1161–6.

[21] Hoermann R, Spoettl G, Berger P, et al. Immunoreactive human chorionic gonadotropin beta core fragment in human pituitary. Exp Clin Endocrinol Diabetes 1995;103:324–31.

[22] Birken S, Maydelman Y, Gawinowicz MA, et al. Isolation and characterization of human pituitary chorionic gonadotropin. Endocrinology 1996;137:1402–11.

[23] Kovaleskaya G, Genbacev O, Fisher SJ, et al. Trophoblast origin of hCG isoforms: cytotrophoblasts are the primary source or choriocarcinoma-like hCG. Mol Cell Endocrinol 2002;194:147–55.

[24] Cole LA, Shahabi S, Oz UA, et al. Hyperglycosylated human chorionic gonadotropin (invasive trophoblast antigen) immunoassay: a new basis for gestational Down syndrome screening. Clin Chem 1999;45:2109–19.

[25] Elliott M, Kardana A, Lustbader JW, et al. Carbohydrate and peptide structure of the α- and β-subunits of human chorionic gonadotropin from normal and aberrant pregnancy and choriocarcinoma. Endocrine 1997;7:15–32.

[26] Cole LA, Khanlian SA, Sutton JM, et al. Hyperglycosylated hCG (invasive trophoblast antigen, ITA) a key antigen for early pregnancy detection. Clin Biochem 2003;36:647–55.

[27] Ozturk M, Berkowitz R, Goldstein D, et al. Differential production of human chorionic gonadotropin and free beta subunits in gestational trophoblastic disease. Am J Obstet Gynecol 1988;158:193–8.

[28] D'Agostino RS, Cole LA, Ponn RB, et al. Urinary gonadotropin fragment in patients with lung and esophageal disease. J Surg Oncol 1992;49:147–50.

[29] Cole LA, Tanaka A, Kim GS, et al. Beta core fragment (β-core / UGF / UGP), a tumor marker: seven year report. Gynecol Oncol 1996;60:264–70.

[30] Marcillac I, Toalen F, Bidart J-M, et al. Free human chorionic gonadotropin β-subunit in gonadal and nongonadal neoplasms. Cancer Res 1992;52:3901–7.

[31] Alfthan H, Haglund C, Roberts P, et al. Elevation of free β-subunit of human choriogonadotropin and core β fragment of choriogonadotropin in serum and urine of patients with malignant pancreatic and biliary disease. Cancer Res 1992;52:4628–33.

[32] Rinne K, Shahabi S, Cole LA. Following metastatic placental site trophoblastic tumor with urine β-core fragment. Gynecol Oncol 1999;74:302–3.

[33] Hoermann R, Spoettl G, Moncayo R, et al. Evidence for the presence of human chorionic gonadotropin (hCG) and free beta-subunit of hCG in the human pituitary. J Clin Endocrinol Metab 1990;71:179–86.

[34] Hancock BW, Newlands ES, Berkowitz RS, et al, editors. Gestational trophoblastic disease. Sheffield: Sheffield University Press; 2003. Available at: www.isstd.org.

[35] Newlands ES. Presentation and management of persistent gestational trophoblastic disease and gestational trophoblastic tumors in the UK. In: Hancock BW, Newland ES, Berkowitz RS, editors. Gestational trophoblastic disease. London: Chapman and Hall; 1997. p. 143–56.

ELSEVIER
SAUNDERS

Obstet Gynecol Clin N Am
32 (2005) 627–640

OBSTETRICS AND
GYNECOLOGY
CLINICS
OF NORTH AMERICA

# Chemotherapeutic Drugs in Pregnancy

## Kimberly K. Leslie, MD*, Christine Koil, MS, William F. Rayburn, MD

*Department of Obstetrics and Gynecology, University of New Mexico Health Sciences Center,
2211 Lomas Boulevard, NE, Albuquerque NM 87131-0001, USA*

Most reproductive-aged women who have cancer are capable of ovulating and, therefore, able to conceive at any time. When pregnancy is diagnosed, chemotherapy may be continued or begun and should not be unnecessarily withheld. In general, systemic therapy for cancer in pregnancy must be individualized and may be different if the patient is diagnosed during the first versus the second or third trimesters. Chemotherapy during the first trimester may cause more severe fetal effects, and in cases where a malignancy that requires chemotherapy is diagnosed during the first trimester, termination of pregnancy is a consideration.

For women who do not request pregnancy termination, the choice of drugs must take into account the fetus and may direct therapy to non-standard regimens (for example, single versus combination therapy). For malignancies diagnosed in the second trimester, consideration for the fetus with respect to drug effects should be given, but in cases of a maternal cancer that responds to chemotherapy, it is unwise to delay treatment until after delivery. Termination of pregnancy is also a possibility, but the effects of the medications on the fetus will potentially be less than in the first trimester.

The likely adverse effects on the fetus have prompted practitioners to consider delaying chemotherapy until the postpartum period for cancers diagnosed in the third trimester. Although it is not prudent to put off definitive treatment for more than a few weeks, it may be possible to effect an early delivery (after steroid therapy to improve fetal lung function and to limit intracranial bleeds) and proceed with chemotherapy in the postpartum period. The University of New

* Corresponding author.
*E-mail address:* kleslie@salud.unm.edu (K.K. Leslie).

Mexico, has offered early delivery for gestations that are past 34 weeks in cases of maternal cancer. At this gestational age, the long-term outcome of a baby approaches that of a term infant. The mother can then receive definitive chemotherapy postpartum without exposing her fetus to potential harm.

## Fetal risks

Physiologic changes of pregnancy must be considered when prescribing chemotherapy. Drugs are easily absorbed, and the serum concentration of albumin for drug binding is lower than when a woman in not pregnant. Pharmacokinetic changes during pregnancy include a higher volume of distribution, lower maximum plasma concentration, lower steady serum state concentration, lower plasma half-life, and higher clearance rate. The small spatial configuration and the high lipid solubility of most chemotherapy facilitate easy transfer of an unbound drug or its metabolite across the placenta or into the breast milk. Virtually all drugs cross the placenta, and therefore, unbound concentrations of the drug are similar or higher in the fetal serum and amniotic fluid than in the maternal serum.

Fetal exposure may be divided into three periods: (1) ovum, from fertilization to implantation; (2) embryo, from the second through the eighth week; and (3) fetus, from the eighth completed week until term. Experience with first trimester exposure for any drug is often too limited in humans to be considered absolutely safe. The embryo period encompasses the most critical time with respect to physical malformations, because it involves organogenesis. The background risks of major defects are about 3% at birth and about 4.5% by 5 years of age.

Despite being infrequent, detrimental effects may occur when certain drugs are taken beyond organogenesis. Few drugs, however, have been implicated in restricting fetal growth or in grossly reducing specific organ size. Of particular importance when prescribing chemotherapy, are the exact dose of the agent and the genetic sensitivity of the mother and fetus. Results of retrospective and uncontrolled studies and individual case reports may be misleading regarding the risk of exposure to specific chemotherapy during pregnancy. Differentiating between effects of a specific pharmacologic agent and effects from an illness can be difficult. There is virtually no information about long-term effects, such as learning or behavior problems (functional teratogenesis), that may result from the chronic prenatal exposure to chemotherapy.

Drugs prescribed during pregnancy have been assigned a risk factor (A, B, C, D, or X) according to definitions provided by the U.S. Food and Drug Administration. Chemotherapeutic agents generally fall into the C or D categories. Drugs in the C category are those for which studies in animals have revealed adverse effects on the fetus (embryocidal, teratogenic, or other) and controlled studies in women or studies in women and animals are not available. Drugs in the D category are those for which there is positive evidence of human fetal risk, but the benefit justifies the potential risk to the fetus. Most human data about chemotherapy during pregnancy involve small series or case reports. Such information may either be biased or merely reflect the patient's background risk for birth defects. Case reports of malformed infants after prenatal exposure to a certain drug, may feature exposures to other agents and a lack of uniformity of abnormalities, which makes their association with a single causative agent unlikely.

## Counseling for pregnancy and breastfeeding

The long-term effect of chemotherapy on female and male reproductive function has been reported for select agents. Menstrual function in most women in regular and premature menopause is very uncommon. Menstrual difficulties are usually not serious or persistent. Problem-free conceptions or, less commonly, initial infertility followed by conception is the norm. We are unaware of any safe minimum time after stopping the drug and conceiving. In addition, spermatogenesis is not impaired long-term. Any infertility requires an assessment of the male factor that includes a sperm count and ejaculate volume.

Treating cancer during pregnancy requires compromises and makes the management of pregnant women who have cancer one of the most challenging areas in all of medicine. This dilemma must take into account the health and welfare of the mother and the fetus, which are at odds when it comes to the use of chemotherapy. Combination therapy is optimal because multiple partially effective drugs used together interrupt a broader range of proliferative pathways that may be pivotal to the growth of individual cells or cell clones. The use of more than one drug is, however, likely to have a greater negative impact on the pregnancy.

A lack of comparability of the dose and the route of administration can also limit interpretation. For example, the short-term administration of a drug given intravenously makes it difficult to relate risk when the same medication is taken orally in a lower dose for a longer period. Because a control population is not possible, it is also difficult to separate any hazard from the medication with that of an underlying disease. Symptoms of pregnancy such as nausea, fatigue, and gastrointestinal disturbance may mimic side effects or toxic reactions to chemotherapy.

Counseling about any harmful risk to the fetus should be performed in a sympathetic, supportive, and informative manner. A detailed targeted ultrasound examination is often used to accurately date the pregnancy and to screen for fetal structural defects. The authors are unaware of any risk of chromosomal abnormalities with chemotherapy before or after conception. For this reason, prenatal genetic testing by first trimester screening, serologic testing, chorionic villus sampling, and amniocentesis, are not recommended. Sources of information regarding potential teratogens include computerized databases online and on diskette. Numerous teratogen information services are available throughout the United States to serve specific geographic areas. Additional sources to which the reader may refer are (1) Chu E, DeVita Jr VT. Cancer chemotherapy drug manual. Sudbury (MA): Jones and Bartlett Publishers; 2005; and (2) Briggs GG, Freeman RK, Yaffe SJ. Drugs in pregnancy and lactation, a reference guide to fetal and neonatal risk. 7th edition. Baltimore (MD):Williams & Wilkins; 2005.

None of the chemotherapeutic agents described here has been proven safe for breastfeeding, and manufacturers recommend breastfeeding be avoided. Contraindications or cautions to breastfeeding are unknown, theoretical, or founded on limited case reports. In general, most medications are excreted in breast milk (often less than 5% of weight adjusted maternal daily doses) leading to legitimate concerns regarding neonatal effects. The amount of drug present in the milk and consumed by the infant depends on the chemical properties of the drug and on the dose, frequency, and duration of exposure. Neonatal neutropenia, immune or bone marrow suppression, and reduced growth are particular concerns with exposure to any chemotherapy.

This article reviews specific effects of commonly used agents by category. For each drug, the literature has been reviewed to provide information on the indication(s), mechanism of action, tissue distribution, maternal and fetal side effects, and breastfeeding information. Information provided in a previous review [1] has been updated and expanded.

## Alkylating agents

Cyclophosphamide (Cytoxin, CTX, CPM, Neosar) is a commonly used agent indicated for breast cancer, non-Hodgkins lymphoma, chronic lymphocytic leukemia, ovarian cancer, bone and soft tissue sarcoma, rhabdomyosarcoma, neuroblastoma, and Wilm's tumor. Cyclophosphamide is also an immunosuppressant and may be indicated for other complications of pregnancy in addition to cancer. The mechanism of action depends upon the fact that cyclophosphamide is activated by the liver cytochrome P450 microsomal system to produce cytotoxic metabolites phosphoramide mustard and acrolein. The metabolites form crosslinks with DNA which results in inhibition of DNA synthesis. This agent is active in all stages of the cell cycle. Cyclophosphamide is distrubuted throughout the body including the brain, cerebrospinal fluid, milk, saliva, and, presumably the amniotic fluid. The drug is given either orally or intravenously, and care providers who administer cyclophosphamide have been reported to absorb measurable quantities of the agent through the skin or air as an aerosol. Women who administer chemotherapy should be aware of this and avoid contact with such drugs during pregnancy [2]. The major maternal side effect is myelosuppression, which is dose-limiting. Normal as well as malformed fetuses have been reported fromexposures during the first trimester [3]. The defects reported include occulofacial malformations, missing digits and nail abnormalities, coronary artery defects, umbilical hernia, hemangioma, imperforate anus, rectovaginal fistula, cleft palate, microcephaly, growth restriction, and developmental delays [3]. Second and third trimester exposures are not associated with malformations, but are linked to growth restriction, microcephaly, and possibly, neonatal pancyto-penia [4]. As with alkylating agents in general, the use of cyclophosphamide is also associated with subsequent menstrual difficulties and premature ovarian failure, although a recent study suggests that successful post-therapy pregnancies are not uncommon [5].

Thiotepa (Triethylenethiophosphoramide, TSPA, Thioplex, Girostan, Tes-pamin, Thiotef) is indicated for the treatment of breast cancer, ovarian cancer, superficial transitional cell cancer of the bladder, and Hodgkins and non-Hodgkin's lymphoma. Thiotepa is an ethylenimine analog that is chemically related to nitrogen mustard, which alkylates the N-7 position of guanine. This damages DNA and inhibits DNA, RNA, and protein synthesis. The drug is active in all phases of the cell cycle and is widely distributed throughout the body including, presumably, the amniotic fluid. Intravenous infusion is required. Little is known about the fetal effects in humans, but thiotepa has been used during the second and third trimesters without apparent harm in one pregnancy [6]. When rats were given high doses of this agent, many of the fetuses died in utero. Multiple malformations are common in surviving pups [7]. In mice, fetal lethality is also a substantial problem, and pups that do not die initially demonstrate a high incidence of skeletal abnormalities when exposed to a mater-nal dose of 5 mg/kg [8].

Chlorambucil (Leukeran) is indicated for the treatment of chronic lymphocytic leukemia and low-grade, non-Hodgkin's lymphoma. Chlorambucil is an analog of nitrogen mustard that cross-links with DNA and inhibits DNA synthesis and function. It is active in all phases of the cell cycle. Chromosomal damage has been documented in human cells following chlorambucil therapy [9]. The drug is given orally, but distribution has not been adequately studied. Myelosuppression is dose-limiting and nadirs at 25–30 days after therapy. As with other alkylating agents, gonadal damage after exposure is a consideration. This raises a concern for premature ovarian failure in women and oligospermia in men [10,11], al-though the agent has been given to patients with recovery of gonadal function and successful pregnancies thereafter [12,13]. Normal pregnancies as well as preg-nancies complicated by fetal malformations have been reported after chlo-rambucil use [14]. Potential effects on the fetus include unilateral agenesis of the left kidney and ureter in male fetuses following first trimester exposure as well as cardiac defects [15,16]. The most consistent finding is renal agenesis in both humans and animals [15–17]; however, the magnitude of the risk in exposed fetuses is not known at this time.

Melphalan (Alkeran, phenylalanine mustard, L-PAM) has been used to treat multiple myeloma, breast cancer, and ovarian cancer. Melphalan is an analog of nitrogen mustard. It forms interstrand and intrastrand cross-links with DNA which results in inhibition of DNA synthesis and function. The drug is active in all phases of the cell cycle and is widely distributed throughout the body including, presumably, the amniotic fluid. It can be given orally or intrave-nously. The principal maternal toxicity is myelosuppression. Ovarian failure and amenorrhea have been reported in women taking melphalan [18,19]. No reports have appeared that link melphalan with congenital defects, although it is possible that this drug has similar effects to other alkylating agents in pregnancy (see cyclophosphomide).

Busulfan (Myleran, Busulfex) is indicated principally for chronic myelogenous leukemia. This is a methanesulfonate-like bifunctional alkylating agent that interacts with thiol groups and causes nucleic acid and protein cross-links. Busulfan is active in all phases of the cell cycle. The drug distributes rapidly in all tissues and crosses into the amniotic fluid and the blood brain barrier. It is given orally or intravenously. Maternal toxicity includes myelosuppression, which is dose-limiting. Rarely, a severe and life threatening form of pulmonary fibrosis results, which may occur 1 to 10 years after therapy. Six of 22 fetuses exposed to busulfan in the first trimester demonstrated malformations including liver and spleen abnormalities, pyloric stenosis, cleft palate, micropthalmia, cytomegaly, hypoplasia of the ovaries and the thyroid, growth restriction, hydronephrosis and absent kidney and ureter [20–22].

Cisplatin (Cis-diamminedechloroplatinum, CDDP, Platinol) is indicated for ovarian cancer, bladder cancer, head and neck cancer, cancer of the esophagus, small cell and non-small cell lung cancer, non-Hodgkin's lymophoma, and choriocarcinoma. Cisplatin covalently binds to DNA preferentially at the N-7 position of guanine and adenine causing cross-links. It also binds to nuclear and cytoplasmic proteins and causes cytotoxic effects. It is widely distributed in all tissues but the highest concentrations occur in the liver and kidneys. The drug is given intravenously or directly into the peritoneal cavity (not absorbed orally). Maternal side effects include nephrotoxicity and neurotoxicity, which are dose-limiting. Myelosuppression is also a factor. Limited use has been reported in pregnancy [23]. There are recent reports of normal neonates born after in utero exposure to a combination of paclitaxel and platinum for ovarian cancer during pregnancy [24,25]. The breastfeeding advice is conflicting. Some references suggest that breastfeeding is possible with caution [26]; however, other references state that breastfeeding should be avoided based upon a report of excretion into breast milk [27].

Carboplatin (Paraplatin, CBDCA) is indicated for ovarian cancer, germ cell tumors, head and neck cancer, small cell and non-small cell lung cancer, bladder cancer, relapsed and refractory acute leukemia, and endometrial cancer. Carboplatin forms DNA cross links preferentially by binding to the N-7 position of guanine and adenine. It is cell cycle non-specific and is widely distributed throughout all body tissues, including presumably, the amniotic fluid. This agent is given intravenously and is not absorbed orally. Maternal myelosuppression is significant and dose-limiting; nephrotoxicity and neurotoxicity are less than with cisplatin. The pregnancy risk category is D; information about fetal effects is limited but likely to be similar to cisplatin. The breastfeeding risks are unknown.

Dacarbazine (DIC, DTIC-Dome, Imidazole carboxamide) is indicated for the treatment of melanoma, Hodgkin's disease, soft tissue sarcomas, and neuroblastoma. Dacarbazine is a non-classical alkylating agent that prevents the biosynthesis of purines. It methylates nucleic acids and inhibits DNA, RNA, and protein synthesis. This agent is distributed throughout the body and fluid spaces. It is loosely bound to plasma proteins. Dacarbazine is given by the intravenous route, and maternal myelosuppression is dose-limiting. Fetal rats exposed to doses ranging from 200 mg to 600 mg demonstrated renal pyelectasis [28]. However, it has been reported that use of dacarbazine in the treatment of metastatic melanoma during the second and third trimester in combination with other medications (carmustine, tamoxifen, and cisplatin) apparently caused no ill-effects. In this case, the baby was delivered prematurely at 30 weeks, but was otherwise healthy [29].

**Antibiotics**

Dactinomycin-D (Actinomycin-D, Act-D, Cosmegen) is indicated for Wilm's tumor, rhabdomyosarcoma, germ cell tumors, gestational trophoblastic disease, and Ewing's sarcoma. Dactinomycin-D is a product of *Streptomyces* species that is composed of a tricyclic phenoxazone chromophore linked to two cyclic polypeptides. This agent binds to guanine-cytidine base pairs and inhibits DNA synthesis and function. It also causes the accumulation of intracellular oxygen-free radicals that further damage DNA. This drug must be given intravenously and is not absorbed orally. Dactinomycin-D concentrates in nucleated blood cells and is highly protein-bound. Maternal myelosuppression is dose-limiting. Reports of the use of dactinomycin-D in the second and third trimesters have revealed apparently normal neonates [10,30–33].

Bleomycin (Blenoxane) is indicated for Hodgkin's disease and non-Hodgkin's lymphoma, germ cell tumors, head and neck cancer, and squamous cell carcinomas of the skin, cervix, and vulva. This drug is a small peptide antibiotic that binds iron to create activated oxygen-free radicals causing breaks in DNA. Bleomycin is given intravenously or directly into the pleural space (not absorbed orally); it is found in the intra and extracellular fluid, where less than 10% is bound to proteins. The major maternal toxicity is pneumonitis, which is dose-limiting. While chromosomal aberrations in human bone marrow cells have been reported [34], no congenital defects have been linked to the use of bleomycin in pregnancy. Second and third trimester exposures in combination with other agents have resulted in the delivery of normal babies [27,31,35,36].

**Antimetabolites**

Methotrexate (MTX, Amethopterin) is indicated for the treatment of breast cancer, head and neck cancer, osteogenic sarcoma, acute lymphocytic leukemia, non-Hodgkin's lymphoma, meningeal leukemia and meningitis, bladder cancer, colorectal cancer, and gestational trophoblastic disease. Methotrexate is a classic folic acid analog/antagonist, and its action is specific for the S-phase of the cell cycle. The drug enters the cell through the folate transport system and inhibits the enzyme dihydrofolate reductase, thus depleting the level of reduced folates necessary for critical cell functions. Methotrexate also inhibits de novo thymidylate and purine synthesis. Upon treatment, it is widely distributed throughout the body including fluid spaces such as the amniotic fluid. The drug is given by the intravenous, intramuscular, or oral routes. Maternal myelosuppression is dose-limiting. Also, acute renal failure caused by intratubular precipitation of methotrexate or its metabolites can occur. In the first trimester, methotrexate is clearly associated with teratogenicity. Malformations include severe cephalic and skull abnormalities with the absence of sutures, absence of the frontal bone, hypertelorism, a depressed or widened nasal bridge, hypoplasia of the mandible, heart defects such as dextroposition, and other conditions including the absence of digits. The attack rate appears to be relatively high; nearly one-third of exposed fetuses demonstrate malformations [37–39]. In addition, late effects of methotrexate on brain development are possible and should be studied further [40].

5-Fluorouracil (5FU, Efudex) is indicated for colorectal cancer, breast cancer, gastrointestinal malignancies, head and neck cancer, skin cancer, hepatoma, and ovarian cancer. This agent is a pyrimidine analog specific for the S-phase of the cell cycle. Metabolic forms are incorporated into DNA and RNA to disrupt cell function. Given intravenously, it is widely distributed in tissues and fluid spaces, including, presumably, the amniotic fluid. Maternal myelosuppression, mucositis, or diarrhea may each be dose-limiting. Hand-foot syndrome, manifested by tingling, skin and nail changes, pain or numbness may also be dose-limiting. Normal as well as malformed fetuses have resulted from exposure to 5-fluorouracil. In one report, first trimester treatment was associated with multiple anomalies including radial dysplasia, absent digits, and hypoplasias of thoracic and abdominal organs such as the lungs, aorta, esophagus, duodenum, and ureters, among other defects [41].

## Nucleoside analogues

Cytarabine (Cytosine arabinoside, Ara-C, Cytosar-U) is indicated for acute myelogenous leukemia, acute lymphocytic leukemia, chronia myelogenous leukemia, and leptomeningeal carcinomatosis. This agent is a deoxycytidine analog synthesized by the sponge *Cryptothethya crypta*. Its activity is specific for the S-phase of the cell cycle where the drug incorporates as a metabolite, ara-C triphosphate, into DNA. This results in the termination of DNA chain synthesis. Intravenous administration results in wide tissue distribution throughout the body including fluid spaces such as the amniotic cavity. The drug is inactive orally. Myelosuppression is dose-limiting for the patient, and the pregnancy risk category is D. First trimester exposures have been associated with otic anomalies and auditory canal atresia, lobster claw hand and other digital anomalies, as well as lower limb defects [42,43]. In addition to the potential for the usual growth restriction in fetuses exposed later in pregnancy, reports of fetal death in utero associated with cytarabine or combinations including cytarabine have appeared in the literature [44]. Breastfeeding data are not available.

Gemcitabine (Gemzar) is indicated for cancer of the pancreas, bladder cancer, non-small cell lung cancer, and soft tissue sarcoma. This drug is a fluorine-substituted deoxycytidine analog that inhibits the cell cycle at the S-phase. Drug exposure results in the incorporation of a metabolic triphosphate nucleotide product, dFdCTP, into DNA that causes chain termination and stops DNA synthesis and function. Gemcitabine is administered by the intravenous route and is not extensively distributed in the body; however, it does cross the blood-brain barrier and may cross the placenta. Maternal myelosuppression is dose-limiting. No information on humans is available at this time; however, gemcitabine is teratogenic in mice and rabbits.

### Topoisomerase I inhibitors

Topotecan (Hycamtin) is indicated for ovarian cancer, small cell lung cancer, and acute myelogenous leukemia. Topotecan is an alkaloid derivative from the *Camptotheca acuminata* tree that inhibits topoisomerase I function. Topotecan binds to and stabilizes the topoisomerase I-DNA complex and prevents the release of DNA after it has been cleaved by topoisomerase I. The complex collides with the advancing replication fork and stops DNA synthesis. This agent is widely distributed in body tissues and is given intravenously. The major maternal toxicity is myelosuppression (dose-limiting) with the neutropenic nadir occurring at 7 – 10 days. No information from humans is available at this time; however, topotecan is teratogenic in animals in dosages that approximate recommended human regimens.

Irinotecan (Camptosar, CPT-II) is indicated for colorectal cancer and non-small cell lung cancer. Irinotecan is a synthetic derivative of camptothecin, an alkaloid derivative of the *Camptotheca acuminata* tree. The active metabolite of irinotecan, SN-38, stabilizes the topoisomerase I-DNA complex and prevents normal DNA synthesis and function. The drug is cell cycle non-specific. This agent is widely distributed throughout the body and is administered intravenously. Myelosuppression is dose-limiting. No studies reporting its use in pregnancy or breastfeeding have appeared.

### Topoisomerase Ii inhibitors

Etoposide (VePesid, VP-16) is indicated for germ cell tumors, small cell lung cancer, non-small cell lung cancer, non-Hodgkin's lymphoma, and gastric cancer. Etoposide is an alkaloid extracted from the *Podophyllum peltatum* mandrake plant that inhibits toposiomerase II by stabilizing the topoisomerase II-DNA complex and preventing DNA unwinding. Etoposide is active during the S- and G2-phases of the cell cycle and is rapidly distributed into all body fluids and tissues when administered either by the intravenous or the oral route. Decreased albumin, as may occur during pregnancy, has the potential to result in elevated free drug levels and toxicity. For the mother, myelosuppression is dose limiting, and etoposide may prolong the prothombin time and the INR. Use of etoposide in pregnancy has not resulted in reported fetal malformations; however, intrauterine growth restriction and pancytopenia in neonates have been reported [45,46]. One child whose mother received etoposide developed ventriculomegaly during the pregnancy and subsequently developed cerebral atrophy [47]; however, most newborns who have been exposed during the second and third trimesters show no abnormalities at two years of development.

Doxorubicin (Adriamycin, Adria, Hydroxydaunorubicin, DOX, Rubex) is indicated for breast cancer, Hodgkin's and non–Hodgkin's lymphoma, soft tissue sarcoma, ovarian cancer, non-small cell and small cell lung cancer, bladder cancer, thyroid cancer, hepatoma, gastric cancer, Wilm's tumor, neuroblastoma, and acute lymphoblastic leukemia. Doxorubicin is an anthracycline antibiotic isolated from *Streptomyces* species that intercalates into DNA, which inhibits DNA synthesis. The drug also inhibits transcription, by inhibiting DNA-dependent RNA polymerase, and the function of topoisomerase II. This agent is widely distributed when given by the intravenous route; about 75% of the drug and metabolites are bound to plasma proteins. Myelosuppression is dose limiting; however, cardiotoxicity, both acute and chronic, are well-described. The acute form presents with arrhythmias and conduction abnormalities and is not dose-related; however, chronic cardiotoxicity is dose-related and results in dilated cardiomyopathy. First trimester exposures, sometimes in combination with other drugs or radiation, have resulted in normal and abnormal neonates. Imperforate anus and rectovaginaol fistula have been described as well as microcephaly [48]. The effects of doxorubicin on the hearts of exposed fetuses and neonates are under evaluation [49], but no definitive information is available. Doxorubicin is excreted in breast milk [50].

Daunorubicin (Daunomycin, DNR, Cerubidine, Rubidomycin) is indicated for acute myelogenous leukemia and acute lymphoblastic leukemia. This drug intercalates into DNA and causes damage by forming a complex between DNA and topoisomerase II. Daunorubicin is widely distributed throughout the major organ systems and is highly lipid soluble. It is given intravenously. Myelosuppression is dose-limiting, and cardiotoxicity is usually transient, but can persist in a chronic form that leads to dilated cardiomyopathy. Fetal effects are presumed to be similar to doxorubicin.

## Vinca alkaloids

Vincristine (Oncovin, VCR) has been used to treat acute lymphoblastic leukemia, Hodgkin's and non-Hodgkin's lymphoma, multiple myeloma, rhabdo-myosarcoma, neuroblastoma, Ewing's sarcoma, Wilm's tumor, chronic leukemias, thyroid cancer, brain tumors, and choriocarcinoma. Vincristine is a vinca

CHEMOTHERAPEUTIC DRUGS IN PREGNANCY       637

alkaloid antimicrotubule agent derived from the periwinkle plant *Catharanthus roseus*. Vincristine inhibits tubulin polymerization and disrupts mitosis; hence this drug is principally active during the M-phase of the cell cycle. This agent is rapidly distributed throughout the body but with relatively poor penetration of the blood-brain barrier; it is given intravenously. Neurotoxicity is dose limiting, and the clinical manifestations include peripheral neuropathy, autonomic nervous system dysfunction, cranial nerve palsies, seizures, cortical blindness, and coma. Various sporadic reports of vincristine use in pregnancy and associated fetal anomalies have appeared. These include the presence of an atrial septal defect, renal hypoplasia, and pancytopenia [4,51,52].

Vinblastine (Velban) has been used to treat Hodgkin's and non-Hodgkin's lymphoma, breast cancer, Kaposi's sarcoma, and renal cell carcinoma. Vinblastine is a plant alkaloid from the periwinkle plant *C. roseus*. It inhibits tubulin polymerization and disrupts microtubules during the M-phase of the cell cycle. It is given intravenously and is widely distributed to most body tissues, but with poor penetration of the blood-brain barrier. Myelosuppression is dose-limiting for the mother, and neurtoxicity is less than with vincristine. Exposure during the first trimester has been associated with normal outcomes [53]; however, a review of cases of vinblastine therapy during pregnancy identified three human cases of suspected teratogenicity. One case was a spontaneous abortion, another resulted in a child with hydrocephalus (first trimester exposure), and another case resulted in the birth of an infant with cleft lip/palate after exposure to a multi-drug regimen including vinblastine [19].

Vinorelbine (Navelbine) may be indicated to treat non-small cell lung cancer, breast cancer, ovarian cancer, and Hodgkin's lymphoma. This agent is a semi-synthetic form of vinblastine with similar actions, which is widely distributed throughout the body and is 80% protein bound. It is given intravenously. Maternal myelosuppression is dose-limiting. Vinorelbine is known to be terato-genic in animals, but sparse data are available in humans.

## Taxanes

Paclitaxel (Taxol) is indicated for the treatment of ovarian cancer, breast cancer, non-small cell and small cell lung cancer, head and neck cancer, esopha-geal cancer, prostate cancer, bladder cancer, endometrial cancer, and AIDS-related Kaposi's sarcoma. Paclitaxel is isolated from the Pacific yew tree, *Taxus brevifolia*. The drug acts by binding to microtubules and enhancing polymeri-zation. Mitosis is inhibited in the M-phase of the cell cycle. This agent is widely distributed throughout the body, including fluid spaces; however, paclitaxel has poor blood brain barrier penetration. It is given by the intravenous route. Myelo-suppression is dose-limiting, and neurotoxocity is a consideration. Rare cases of fatal anaphylaxis have been reported. A few case reports of human fetal exposures have appeared in the literature. These include one patient who was treated from 16 weeks until delivery; the baby was reported to be normal at

15 months [24], and another patient who was treated from 27 weeks until delivery; the baby was a normal neonate when evaluated at 30 months of age [25]. Paclitaxel is highly lipophilic, and minimal kinetic information is available.

## Biologics and growth factor pathway blocking agents

Trastuzumab (Herceptin) is one of a new class of anti-cancer therapies that block the epidermal growth factor receptor (EGFR) pathway. Specifically, trastuzumab blocks the HER-2/neu receptor, a member of the EGFR family. This agent has shown promise in the treatment of breast and lung cancer and is in trials for treatment of endometrial and ovarian cancer, among other sites. It has now gained approval from the Food and Drug Administration for the treatment of advanced breast cancer. Interestingly, the manufacturer has assigned a pregnancy risk category of B to trastuzumab based upon extensive trials in monkeys without apparent fetal harm. Placental transfer in monkeys was demonstrated. However, a case report of the use of trastuzumab in human pregnancy reveals an association with significantly decreased amniotic fluid, indicating an adverse effect on the fetal kidney [54]. In addition, mice in which the HER-2/neu gene has been deleted, die during embryogenesis because of heart defects or lack of proper cardiac development [55]. These reports indicate that biologics, as well as classic chemotherapy agents, have the potential to affect the fetus and should be used with caution for the treatment of cancer in pregnancy.

## References

[1] Leslie KK. Chemotherapy and pregnancy. Clin Obstet Gynecol 2002;45(1):153–64.
[2] Hirst M, Tse S, Mills DG, et al. Occupational exposure to cyclophosphamide. Lancet 1984; 1(8370):186–8.
[3] Enns GM, Roeder E, Chan RT, et al. Apparent cyclophosphamide (cytoxan) embryopathy: a distinct phenotype? Am J Med Genet 1999;86(3):237–41.
[4] Pizzuto J, Aviles A, Noriega L, et al. Treatment of acute leukemia during pregnancy: presentation of nine cases. Cancer Treat Rep 1980;64(4–5):679–83.
[5] Yoshinaka A, Fukasawa I, Sakamoto T, et al. The fertility and pregnancy outcomes of the patients who underwent preservative operation followed by adjuvant chemotherapy for malignant ovarian tumors. Arch Gynecol Obstet 2000;264(3):124–7.
[6] Dobbing J. Pregnancy and leukaemia. Lancet 1977;1(8022):1155.
[7] Murphy ML, Del Moro A, Lacon C. The comparative effects of five polyfunctional alkylating agents on the rat fetus, with additional notes on the chick embryo. Ann N Y Acad Sci 1958;68(3):762–81 [discussion 781–62].
[8] Korogodina Iu V, Kaurov BA. Teratogenic effect of thiophosphamide on mice of different genotypes. Byull Eksp Biol Med 1984;97(3):331–2.
[9] van der Steen J, van Wichen BH, Benckhuysen C. Effects of alkylating agents on the DNA replication of cultured Yoshida sarcoma cells. Chem Biol Interact 1982;39(2):191–204.
[10] Freckman HA, Fry HL, Mendez FL, et al. Chlorambucil-prednisolone therapy for disseminated breast carcinoma. JAMA 1964;189:23–6.

[11] Morgenfeld MC, Goldberg V, Parisier H, et al. Ovarian lesions due to cytostatic agents during the treatment of Hodgkin's disease. Surg Gynecol Obstet 1972;134(5):826–8.

[12] Callis L, Nieto J, Vila A, et al. Chlorambucil treatment in minimal lesion nephrotic syndrome: a reappraisal of its gonadal toxicity. J Pediatr 1980;97(4):653–6.

[13] Richter P, Calamera JC, Morgenfeld MC, et al. Effect of chlorambucil on spermatogenesis in the human with malignant lymphoma. Cancer 1970;25(5):1026–30.

[14] Jacobs C, Donaldson SS, Rosenberg SA, et al. Management of the pregnant patient with Hodgkin's disease. Ann Intern Med 1981;95(6):669–75.

[15] Shotton D, Monie IW. Possible teratogenic effect of chlorambucil on a human fetus. JAMA 1963;186:74–5.

[16] Steege JF, Caldwell DS. Renal agenesis after first trimester exposure to chlorambucil. South Med J 1980;73(10):1414–5.

[17] Kavlock RJ, Rehnberg BF, Rogers EH. Chlorambucil induced congenital renal hypoplasia: effects on basal renal function in the developing rat. Toxicology 1986;40(3):247–58.

[18] Rose DP, Davis TE. Ovarian function in patients receiving adjuvant chemotherapy for breast cancer. Lancet 1977;1(8023):1174–6.

[19] Schilsky RL, Lewis BJ, Sherins RJ, et al. Gonadal dysfunction in patients receiving chemotherapy for cancer. Ann Intern Med 1980;93(1):109–14.

[20] Lee RA, Johnson CE, Hanlon DG. Leukemia during pregnancy. Am J Obstet Gynecol 1962;84: 455–8.

[21] Diamond I, Anderson MM, Mc Creadie SR. Transplacental transmission of busulfan (myleran) in a mother with leukemia. Production of fetal malformation and cytomegaly. Pediatrics 1960; 25:85–90.

[22] Abramovici A, Shaklai M, Pinkhas J. Myeloschisis in a six weeks embryo of a leukemic woman treated by busulfan. Teratology 1978;18(2):241–6.

[23] Marana HR, de Andrade JM, da Silva Mathes AC, et al. Chemotherapy in the treatment of locally advanced cervical cancer and pregnancy. Gynecol Oncol 2001;80(2):272–4.

[24] Mendez LE, Mueller A, Salom E, et al. Paclitaxel and carboplatin chemotherapy administered during pregnancy for advanced epithelial ovarian cancer. Obstet Gynecol 2003;102(5 Pt 2): 1200–2.

[25] Sood AK, Shahin MS, Sorosky JI. Paclitaxel and platinum chemotherapy for ovarian carcinoma during pregnancy. Gynecol Oncol 2001;83(3):599–600.

[26] American Academy of Pediatrics Committee on Drugs. The transfer of drugs and other chemicals into human milk. Pediatrics 1994;93(1):137–50.

[27] de Vries EG, van der Zee AG, Uges DR, et al. Excretion of platinum into breast milk. Lancet 1989;1(8636):497.

[28] Chaube S, Swinyard CA. Urogenital anomalies in fetal rats produced by the anticancer agent 4(5)-(3,3-dimethyl-1-triazeno) imidazole-4-carboxamide. Anat Rec 1976;186(3):461–9.

[29] Dipaola RS, Goodin S, Ratzell M, et al. Chemotherapy for metastatic melanoma during pregnancy. Gynecol Oncol 1997;66(3):526–30.

[30] Gililland J, Weinstein L. The effects of cancer chemotherapeutic agents on the developing fetus. Obstet Gynecol Surv 1983;38(1):6–13.

[31] Haerr RW, Pratt AT. Multiagent chemotherapy for sarcoma diagnosed during pregnancy. Cancer 1985;56(5):1028–33.

[32] Weed JC, Roh RA, Mendenhall HW. Recurrent endodermal sinus tumor during pregnancy. Obstet Gynecol 1979;54(5):653–6.

[33] Kim DS, Park MI. Maternal and fetal survival following surgery and chemotherapy of endodermal sinus tumor of the ovary during pregnancy: a case report. Obstet Gynecol 1989;73(3 Pt 2): 503–7.

[34] Bornstein RS, Hungerford DA, Haller G, et al. Cytogenetic effects of bleomycin therapy in man. Cancer Res 1971;31(12):2004–7.

[35] Ortega J. Multiple agent chemotherapy including bleomycin of non-Hodgkin's lymphoma during pregnancy. Cancer 1977;40(6):2829–35.

[36] Falkson HC, Simson IW, Falkson G. Non-Hodgkin's lymphoma in pregnancy. Cancer 1980; 45(7):1679–82.

[37] Milunsky A, Graef JW, Gaynor Jr MF. Methotrexate-induced congenital malformations. J Pediatr 1968;72(6):790–5.

[38] Powell HR, Ekert H. Methotrexate-induced congenital malformations. Med J Aust 1971;2(21): 1076–7.

[39] Warkany J. Teratogenicity of folic acid antagonists. Cancer Bull 1981;33:76–7.

[40] MacDougall MK, LeGrand SB, Walsh D. Symptom control in the pregnant cancer patient. Semin Oncol 2000;27(6):704–11.

[41] Stephens JD, Golbus MS, Miller TR, et al. Multiple congenital anomalies in a fetus exposed to 5-fluorouracil during the first trimester. Am J Obstet Gynecol 1980;137(6):747–9.

[42] Wagner VM, Hill JS, Weaver D, et al. Congenital abnormalities in baby born to cytarabine treated mother. Lancet 1980;2(8185):98–9.

[43] Schafer AI. Teratogenic effects of antileukemic chemotherapy. Arch Intern Med 1981;141(4): 514–5.

[44] Volkenandt M, Buchner T, Hiddemann W, et al. Acute leukaemia during pregnancy. Lancet 1987;2(8574):1521–2.

[45] Buller RE, Darrow V, Manetta A, et al. Conservative surgical management of dysgerminoma concomitant with pregnancy. Obstet Gynecol 1992;79(5 Pt 2):887–90.

[46] Murray NA, Acolet D, Deane M, et al. Fetal marrow suppression after maternal chemotherapy for leukaemia. Arch Dis Child Fetal Neonatal Ed 1994;71(3):F209–10.

[47] Elit L, Bocking A, Kenyon C, et al. An endodermal sinus tumor diagnosed in pregnancy: case report and review of the literature. Gynecol Oncol 1999;72(1):123–7.

[48] Murray CL, Reichert JA, Anderson J, et al. Multimodal cancer therapy for breast cancer in the first trimester of pregnancy. A case report. JAMA 1984;252(18):2607–8.

[49] Meyer-Wittkopf M, Barth H, Emons G, et al. Fetal cardiac effects of doxorubicin therapy for carcinoma of the breast during pregnancy: case report and review of the literature. Ultrasound Obstet Gynecol 2001;18(1):62–6.

[50] Egan PC, Costanza ME, Dodion P, et al. Doxorubicin and cisplatin excretion into human milk. Cancer Treat Rep 1985;69(12):1387–9.

[51] Thomas PR, Biochem D, Peckham MJ. The investigation and management of Hodgkin's disease in the pregnant patient. Cancer 1976;38(3):1443–51.

[52] Mennuti MT, Shepard TH, Mellman WJ. Fetal renal malformation following treatment of Hodgkin's disease during pregnancy. Obstet Gynecol 1975;46(2):194–6.

[53] Garrett MJ. Teratogenic effects of combination chemotherapy. Ann Intern Med 1974; 80(5):667 [letter].

[54] Watson WJ. Herceptin (trastuzumab) therapy during pregnancy: association with reversible anhydramnios. Obstet Gynecol 2005;105(3):642–3.

[55] Lee KF, Simon H, Chen H, et al. Requirement for neuregulin receptor erbB2 in neural and cardiac development. Nature 1995;378(6555):394–8.

ELSEVIER
SAUNDERS

Obstet Gynecol Clin N Am
32 (2005) 641–660

OBSTETRICS AND
GYNECOLOGY
CLINICS
OF NORTH AMERICA

# Gastrointestinal, Pancreatic, and Hepatic Cancer During Pregnancy

Jeffrey C. Dunkelberg, MD, PhD[a],*, Jehad Barakat, MD[a],
John Deutsch, MD[b]

[a]Division of Gastroenterology and Hepatology, Department of Internal Medicine,
University of New Mexico Health Sciences Center, Ambulatory Care Center-5,
1 University of New Mexico, MSC10-5550, Albuquerque, NM 87131–0001, USA
[b]Division of Gastroenterology, St. Mary's Duluth Clinic, 400 East Third Street,
Duluth, MN 55805, USA

Pregnancy affects the clinical presentation, evaluation, treatment, and prognosis of patients with gastrointestinal cancer. Pregnant patients may present with advanced gastrointestinal cancer as a result of delayed diagnosis, in part because of difficulty differentiating signs and symptoms of cancer from signs and symptoms of normal pregnancy. The approach to cancer surgery and chemotherapy must be modified in pregnant patients to minimize fetal and maternal risks, depending on the stage of gestation. Because of these factors, women who develop gastrointestinal cancers during pregnancy seem to have a poor prognosis. This article focuses on cancers of the colon, stomach, pancreas, and liver that occur during pregnancy.

## Colorectal cancer

*Incidence*

Colorectal cancer is the second most common cause of cancer death in women [1]. Only 4% to 8% of colorectal cancers, however, occur in patients less than 40 years of age [2,3]. The mean age of pregnant patients with colorectal cancer in

* Corresponding author.
*E-mail address:* jdunkelberg@salud.unm.edu (J.C. Dunkelberg).

0889-8545/05/$ – see front matter. Published by Elsevier Inc.
doi:10.1016/j.ogc.2005.08.004                    *obgyn.theclinics.com*

a large review was 31 years (range, 16–48 years) [4]. The incidence of colon cancer during pregnancy is estimated to be 1 in 13,000 [5]; up to 300 of the approximate 4 million pregnancies per year in the United States are complicated by colorectal cancer. According to Cappell [6], about 300 cases of colorectal cancer during pregnancy have been reported.

*Risk factors*

High-risk groups for colorectal cancer include patients with familial adenomatous polyposis coli [7], hereditary nonpolyposis colorectal cancer syndrome [8], long-standing inflammatory bowel disease [9], and those with an extensive family history of colon cancer [8]. These high-risk groups account for a small minority (5%–10%) of all colorectal cancer cases, but are more likely to be present in younger patients, including those in the age cohort in which pregnancies occur. In two studies of a total of 24 pregnant patients with colorectal cancer, 6 had risk factors of ulcerative colitis or adenomatous polyposis coli [10,11]. Because colon cancers in high-risk patients often occur before the age of 40 years, these individuals at higher risk should have periodic colonoscopies beginning at a young age [12]. Women with a history of ulcerative colitis or Crohn's colitis for more than 10 years should undergo surveillance colonoscopy every 1 to 2 years with random mucosal biopsies collected to look for dysplasia. Finally, consideration should be given to elective screening, or evaluation of symptoms that could be related to colorectal neoplasia, in high-risk individuals before pregnancy.

*Presentation*

Symptoms of colorectal cancer include abdominal pain, rectal bleeding, nausea, vomiting, abdominal distention, and constipation [5,6,11,13]. Anemia, caused by a combination of gastrointestinal bleeding and the physiologic anemia of pregnancy [14], may produce weakness, fatigue, and pallor. Abdominal pain, nausea, vomiting, and hypoactive or high-pitched bowel sounds suggest gastrointestinal obstruction. Colonic perforation from colon cancer is more common during pregnancy [15]; signs suggestive of colonic perforation include fever, abdominal rebound tenderness, and hypoactive bowel sounds. Rectal examination may detect rectal cancers and fecal occult blood testing may be positive.

Diagnostic evaluation of symptoms from colon cancer in pregnancy may be delayed because some of these symptoms are common in pregnancy and colon cancer may not be considered as a potential problem in a young pregnant patient. Pregnancy can cause altered bowel habits, abdominal pain, abdominal swelling, nausea, vomiting, and anemia. The differential diagnosis of rectal bleeding in a pregnant patient includes hemorrhoids, ulcerative colitis, Crohn's disease, infectious colitis, and colorectal cancer.

*Diagnosis*

*Abdominal imaging*

Abdominal CT is usually performed to detect local extension or metastases in the nonpregnant patient with colorectal cancer, but is contraindicated during pregnancy, especially during the first trimester, because of radiation teratogenicity [16]. Abdominal ultrasound is the procedure of choice to evaluate the liver during pregnancy [17]. Ultrasound is relatively sensitive, with an overall 75% rate of detection of hepatic metastases [18]. Ultrasound is highly sensitive for metastatic liver lesions greater than 2 cm in diameter, but is much less sensitive for metastatic lesions less than 1 cm in diameter.

*Sigmoidoscopy and colonoscopy*

The most accurate method to diagnose colorectal cancer involves endoscopy, either using a short (65 cm) instrument (sigmoidoscopy) or a long (160 cm) instrument (colonoscopy). In the general population, only 20% to 25% of colon cancers occur in the rectum [1,19], which for all practical purposes is the distal 10 to 15 cm of the colon. A recent Veterans Administration cooperative study suggested that 65% of colorectal cancers in average-risk women occur in the proximal colon beyond the reach of the standard sigmoidoscope [20]. In contrast, most reported colorectal cancers in pregnant patients have occurred in the rectum. Bernstein and coworkers [4] reviewed the published literature for 205 cases of colorectal cancer during pregnancy and found that 86% were located in the rectum. These investigators also reported their own experience with colorectal cancer during pregnancy; 64% of cancers were rectal and 36% were colonic [4]. The rectal predominance of colorectal cancer during pregnancy may result from increased detection because of frequent pelvic and rectal examinations, or exacerbation of rectal symptoms caused by rectal compression by the gravid uterus [4].

The fetal safety and clinical efficacy of gastrointestinal endoscopy during pregnancy has recently been reviewed by Cappell [21]. Sigmoidoscopy is indicated during pregnancy to evaluate rectal bleeding and for evaluation of a suspected rectosigmoid stricture or mass. Sigmoidoscopy has not been reported to induce labor or result in congenital malformations [21–23]. In a case-controlled study of 46 patients undergoing sigmoidoscopy during pregnancy, there was no increased incidence of poor pregnancy outcome and Apgar scores were not significantly different from the national mean [6,22].

In nonpregnant patients, complete colonoscopy is indicated for evaluation of rectal bleeding, hemoccult-positive stools, change in bowel habits, and obstructive symptoms. Complete colonoscopy is necessary preoperatively in nonpregnant patients diagnosed with colorectal cancer for pathologic diagnosis and for excluding synchronous colonic lesions (which occur in 5% of colorectal cancer patients) [24,25]. Sigmoidoscopy may be preferred initially during pregnancy, however, because no sedation is required.

In contrast to sigmoidoscopy, the safety of colonoscopy during pregnancy is not as well established [6,21]. Theoretical risks from colonoscopy during

pregnancy include placental abruption, teratogenicity from endoscopic medications, and fetal toxicity from intraprocedural maternal hypotension or hypoxia
[6,21]. In a study of eight colonoscopies during pregnancy, excluding one volun-
tary elective abortion, six of seven pregnant patients delivered healthy babies
after colonoscopy [22]. The patient who did not suffered a miscarriage associated
with severe colorectal bleeding caused by severe ulcerative colitis 4 months after
colonoscopy. As reviewed by Cappell [6], in seven other published case reports
of colonoscopy during pregnancy, the fetal outcomes included three healthy
preterm babies; one healthy full-term baby; two still-births, neither temporally
related to the colonoscopy [5,6,11,26,27]; and one unknown outcome [28].

Colonoscopy may be necessary during pregnancy for evaluation of bleeding
or obstructive symptoms, and before colon cancer surgery to obtain a pathologic
diagnosis and to exclude synchronous colonic lesions. For procedural conscious
sedation in pregnant patients, meperidine has a documented fetal safety profile
[21], and limiting meperidine dosage to 75 mg or less to avoid fetal oversedation
is recommended [21,29]. Propofol, administered by an anesthesiologist, is also
safe for use in pregnant patients in the second and third trimesters, although its
safety in the first trimester has not been studied [21,30,31]. Fetal cardiac
monitoring should be considered to detect intraprocedural fetal distress during
endoscopic procedures for pregnant patients.

*Transrectal ultrasonography*

Transrectal endoscopic ultrasonography helps stage rectal cancer preoperatively; however, it has not been evaluated in pregnant patients. Rectal ultrasonography could be especially helpful in late pregnancy to determine whether a
large and anterior rectal cancer could compress the cervix and preclude vaginal
delivery [6].

*Barium enema*

Barium enema is contraindicated in pregnancy because of potential radiation
teratogenicity [16].

*Therapy*

*Pathologic stage*

Therapy for colon cancer is dependant on tumor stage. Colon cancer is most
commonly staged using the TNM (*T*umor, *N*odes, *M*etastases) classification, with
stages from I to IV. Stage I colorectal cancer is confined to the muscularis
propria; stage II invades through the muscularis propria, but with no lymph nodes
involved by tumor; stage III has regional lymph node metastases; and stage IV
has distant metastases. Pathologic stage is highly correlated with cancer prognosis [32].

Difficulties diagnosing colorectal cancer during pregnancy may explain the
reported high frequency of advanced pathologic cancer stage in these patients. Of

39 colorectal cancers during pregnancy reviewed by Bernstein and coworkers [4], 60% had metastases to either lymph nodes or distant organs.

*Surgery*

Surgery is the primary therapy for colorectal cancer during pregnancy [6,33,34]. The type and timing of surgery depends on gestational age, colorectal cancer stage, maternal cancer prognosis, intraoperative findings, and maternal desires.

When colorectal cancer is diagnosed during the first half of pregnancy, cancer surgery should be promptly performed to minimize the risk of metastases [35]. Surgery during the first half of pregnancy can be performed without removing the gravid uterus [4]. Total abdominal hysterectomy, however, may be necessary to facilitate access to the rectum when needed for intraoperative exposure, when the mother's predicted survival is less than the time needed for the fetus to become viable, or when the cancer extends into the uterus [11,36]. Otherwise, when the cancer appears resectable, curative surgery should be performed leaving the pregnancy intact. When the cancer is unresectable, a colostomy can be performed for cancer palliation until the fetus becomes viable.

When colorectal cancer is diagnosed during the second half of pregnancy, cancer surgery should be delayed until the fetus is viable, at which time vaginal delivery should be induced [6,33]. Cancer resection should be delayed for several days postpartum to permit involution of the uterus and resolution of pelvic vascular congestion [11], although prolonged delay permits cancer growth and metastases [11,35].

Because of a high incidence of ovarian metastases during pregnancy, Nesbitt and colleagues [11] recommend routine intraoperative bilateral ovarian wedge biopsies with pathologic analysis of frozen sections. Bilateral salpingo-oophorectomy is indicated when the ovaries are involved or when hysterectomy is required [11,34].

Delivery by cesarean section is performed for the same obstetric indications as in patients without colon cancer [6]. Cesarean section is also indicated when a large rectal cancer compresses the birth canal or is located anteriorly, because birth trauma or an episiotomy could result in entering into the cancer [34,37]. Colorectal cancer surgery can be performed when cesarean section is performed.

*Chemotherapy*

Chemotherapy for colon cancer has changed markedly in the past several years. Previously, the standard chemotherapeutic agent for advanced colorectal carcinoma was 5-fluorouracil. Subsequently, the Food and Drug Administration has approved two drugs for use as first-line agents (oxiliplatin and irinotecan), and more recently, two biologic agents have been approved (bevacizumab and cetuximab) [38].

Adjuvant therapy (therapy given after an apparent surgical cure) with 5-fluorouracil–containing regimens has been shown to improve survival in stage III and in some cases of stage II colorectal cancer [39]. There are no reports of a live birth following first-trimester exposure to 5-fluorouracil [34]. If a woman with stage III colorectal cancer diagnosed early in pregnancy is treated with curative surgery and elects to consider adjuvant chemotherapy, she needs to be informed of the potential effects of 5-fluorouracil on the fetus during the early stages of pregnancy.

Chemotherapy is safer when administered during the second or third trimester, with no increase in fetal loss or developmental abnormalities [11,40]. There is, however, a significant increase in the incidence of intrauterine growth retardation and prematurity with adjuvant chemotherapy [6,34]. Adjuvant chemotherapy could be used late in pregnancy in a patient who has undergone colorectal resection early in pregnancy, although the benefit of adjuvant chemotherapy for stage III colorectal cancer has not been determined when delayed more than 6 weeks from surgical resection [39]. Delaying adjuvant chemotherapy until after delivery could be considered for stage III colorectal cancer diagnosed late in pregnancy.

### Radiotherapy

Preoperative or postoperative radiotherapy decreases the risk of local rectal cancer recurrence and increases survival [41]. Pelvic radiation for rectal cancer is contraindicated during pregnancy, however, and can be used only after delivery or termination of pregnancy.

### Prognosis

### Maternal prognosis

Maternal outcomes for rectal cancer diagnosed during pregnancy have been relatively poor; the 5-year disease-free survival was only 42% in a study of 26 pregnant patients with rectal cancer [4]. The prognosis for colon cancer above the rectum may be worse [4,11]. Nesbitt and coworkers [11] reported no 5-year survivors among 23 patients with colon cancer during pregnancy. The poor maternal outcome for colorectal cancer in pregnancy may result from the high incidence of advanced pathologic stage at diagnosis [11]. When stratified according to pathologic stage, the 5-year cancer survival in pregnant patients is no different than in the general population [4].

Human chorionic gonadotropin production by colorectal cancers may be associated with a poor prognosis [42] and, importantly, a positive test for β human chorionic gonadotropin in a young woman with colon cancer does not always indicate pregnancy [43]. Gastrointestinal tumors, particularly colon cancers, may produce human chorionic gonadotropin [43–45]. Serum β human chorionic gonadotropin is detectable in 5% to 41% of colorectal cancer patients [44,46], whereas immunohistochemical studies have demonstrated the presence of immunoreactive β human chorionic gonadotropin in tumor cells in 43% to 52% of colorectal cancers [45–47]. The presence of β human chorionic gonadotropin in colonic cancer is reported to be associated with mucinous adenocarcinoma, poorly differentiated adenocarcinoma, a greater degree of local invasion, and the presence of metastases [45].

Ovarian metastases are associated with a poor prognosis [48–51]. The incidence of colon cancer metastases to the ovary in nonpregnant women is approximately 25% in women less than 40 years of age [50–52]. Case reports suggest that pregnant patients have a similar high incidence of ovarian metastases [11,53].

*Fetal prognosis*

Colon cancer rarely produces placental metastases (one report) [54] and has not been reported to cause fetal metastases [6]. Fetal morbidity and mortality seem to relate to maternal factors and therapy-related complications.

Limited data exist on fetal outcome following colon cancer surgery early in pregnancy because colon cancer has rarely been detected before 20 weeks of gestation [4]. A few healthy infants have been born after colorectal surgery early in pregnancy, including abdominoperineal resection [18,28]. The rate of fetal death after major intra-abdominal or extra-abdominal surgery is 3.8% [55], with no postoperative fetal deaths in a study of 60 laparotomies, as compared with a 2% rate of fetal death in pregnant controls not undergoing surgery. Laparotomy, however, is associated with a high risk of preterm delivery and low birth weight [55]. Kort and coworkers [55] reported a premature delivery rate of 21.8% after major surgery, about twice the rate in pregnant controls. Tocolytics are usually administered to prevent spontaneous abortion from postoperative uterine contractions [55].

Although the fetal prognosis from maternal colon cancer is relatively favorable, infant mortality is still about 20% [5,11,56]. Fetal deaths are most commonly caused by prematurity, although stillbirth and spontaneous abortion also occur. In one series [56], 69% of live-born infants had birth weights under 2500 g.

## Gastric cancer during pregnancy

*Incidence*

Gastric cancer is most frequent in middle-aged and elderly populations (mean age 60 years) and is unusual in individuals younger than 40 years [57,58]. Only 3.5% to 6.5% of gastric cancer patients are less than age 40 [57,59]. Overall, gastric cancer is more common in men than women, with a ratio of 1.7:1 [60], but the male-to-female ratio shows a predominance of females in the younger population (1:1–1:2.5) [59,61]. The frequency of gastric cancer during pregnancy seems to be highest in Japan, where 200 to 300 pregnant women (about 0.026%) per year are likely to have gastric cancer [62]. Most of the literature concerning gastric cancer in pregnancy has been based on Japanese patients and the Japanese experience.

There are three relatively large series analyzing patients with gastric cancer during pregnancy [59,63,64]. In 1991, Ueo and coworkers [64] reviewed the Japanese literature and noted reports of 104 cases of gastric cancer during pregnancy. These investigators also reviewed 61 Japanese cases diagnosed between 1968 and 1988. In 1999, Jaspers and coworkers [63] analyzed 92 cases of gastric cancer in pregnancy, 61 of which were from the Japanese literature, and another 31 from the non-Japanese literature. In both series, about one third of cases were detected before 30 weeks gestation, one third after 30 weeks, and one third detected after delivery. Nearly all tumors were found in advanced stages; two cases of early cancer were identified in Japan. Most showed poorly differentiated and diffuse type histology.

The third series of gastric cancer during pregnancy was reported by Maeta and co-workers in 1995 [59]. Pregnancy-associated gastric cancers were defined as cases of gastric cancer detected during pregnancy and cases in which the interval between the initiation of pregnancy and the diagnosis of gastric cancer was less than 2 years. A total of 2325 consecutive Japanese patients with gastric cancer who attended a single clinic were reviewed from the 25 years between 1966 and 1990. Fourteen pregnancy-associated cases of gastric cancer were identified, four diagnosed during pregnancy. Overall, for patients less than 40 years, the male to female ratio was 1:1.7, and was 1:2 for the population of patients less than 30 years. The 14 pregnancy-associated cases comprised 14.7% of the total of 95 women less than 40 years of age with gastric cancer. The mean age of the pregnancy-associated gastric cancer patients was 31.4 (range, 26–37 years). The mean interval between the initiation of pregnancy and the diagnosis of gastric cancer was 14.6 months (range, 2–22 months), with four diagnosed during pregnancy.

*Risk factors*

Gastric cancer occurs more commonly in populations outside of North America, with Japan having a relatively high incidence [65]. Dietary factors, such as salt preservation of food, may contribute to gastric cancer risk [65]. Infection with *Helicobacter pylori* is another potential risk factor that recent data suggest may be more important in women than men [66].

*Presentation*

The diagnosis of gastric cancer in pregnancy may be difficult, because symptoms of the carcinoma may be misinterpreted as pregnancy-induced nausea and discomfort. Early gastric cancer is generally asymptomatic. Symptoms of more advanced gastric cancer include nausea, vomiting, epigastric pain, anorexia, abdominal distention, and fullness of the stomach [64]. Nausea and vomiting during pregnancy is common, however, affecting between 50% and 90% of gravidas. Vomiting ceases by the sixteenth week in approximately 90% of patients, and by the twentieth week in 99% [67]. Significant nausea and vomiting that persists into the second half of pregnancy should not be regarded as normal and diagnostic testing should be considered.

## Diagnosis

Upper endoscopy is a sensitive method for detecting gastric cancer. Upper endoscopy should be performed for patients with persistent epigastric complaints in the second trimester, especially if associated with signs of upper gastrointestinal bleeding, weight loss, or in the absence of appropriate weight gain [59,63,64].

The fetal safety and clinical efficacy of upper gastrointestinal endoscopy during pregnancy has been recently reviewed by Cappell [21]. Clinical studies indicate that the benefits of upper endoscopy exceed the risks when performed for overt gastrointestinal bleeding. Upper endoscopy is also indicated for severe refractory nausea and vomiting accompanied by significant abdominal pain, hematemesis, or signs of gastroduodenal obstruction. Endoscopic ultrasonography may be useful to stage the local extent and regional lymph node involvement of gastric cancer, although there are no reports using this modality during pregnancy.

## Therapy

### Surgery

Practical guidelines for treatment of gastric cancer during pregnancy are similar to those for colorectal cancer during pregnancy [64]. The management of gastric cancer during pregnancy is determined by both the gestational age of the fetus and the stage of the tumor. If complications, such as hemorrhage, obstruction, or perforation, are present, immediate surgery without delay is mandatory at any stage of pregnancy.

Ueo and coworkers developed a treatment algorithm [64] that has been accepted by other reviewers of gastric cancer during pregnancy [63,68]. These investigators divided patients with gastric cancer during pregnancy into four groups, depending on gestational age at the time of gastric cancer diagnosis. In group I patients, the gastric cancer is diagnosed before the twenty-fourth gestational week when the recommendation is "surgical treatment for gastric cancer should be immediately performed without regard for the pregnancy" [64]. In group II patients, gastric cancer is diagnosed between the twenty-fifth to twenty-ninth gestational week. The treatment decision at this interval depends on the stage of gastric cancer. If the cancer is advanced and considered resectable, immediate resection of the gastric cancer is recommended despite the risk to the fetus. If the gastric cancer is early, treatment may be postponed until the thirtieth gestational week to ensure safer delivery. In group III patients, the gastric cancer is diagnosed after the thirtieth week of gestation when cesarean section or vaginal delivery is applicable. The recommended approach is delivery when the infant is viable, followed by a radical operation for the gastric cancer. In group IV patients, gastric cancer is diagnosed after delivery, when the pregnancy has little impact on treatment decisions.

Laparotomy was performed in 47 cases (77.1%) in the Ueo series [64]. Fourteen patients (23%) were not candidates for surgery because of either poor physical condition or highly advanced cancer. Surgical resection of the gastric cancer was achieved in 29 cases (47.5%). In the resected cases, 9 underwent total gastrectomy, 7 subtotal gastrectomy, and 13 partial gastrectomy.

*Chemotherapy*

In the past, adjuvant chemotherapy for gastric cancer has not been as efficacious as it has been for colorectal cancer. Recently, however, adjuvant chemoradiotherapy has been shown to improve survival in patients with gastric cancer [69,70]. Consideration should be given to using adjuvant therapy for gastric cancer during pregnancy with the same caveats in timing of treatment as discussed for colon cancer.

*Prognosis*

In the general population, survival from gastric cancer is poor. In the review by Dupont and coworkers [71], the 5-year survival rate for all ages ranged from 5.1% to 12%, with an average of 7.3% in series of greater than 1000 patients.

Similarly, the prognosis for patients with gastric cancer diagnosed during pregnancy is poor [59,63,64]. Overall, 88% of patients die within 1 year. Of 61 Japanese patients analyzed by Ueo and coworkers [64], 96.7% were in an advanced stage at the time of diagnosis. Only two cases of early cancer were noted. The incidence of hospital death was high: 58.9% overall, 92.9% in inoperable cases, 57.1% in surgically treated patients, and 22.7% after gastrectomy. The incidence of in-hospital death was higher when the gastric cancer was diagnosed during gestation than when diagnosed in the postpartum period. Of resected cases, 31.6% survived 1 year, 21.1% survived 3 years, and 5.3% survived 4 years. All of the unresected cases died within 6 months of detection of the gastric cancer. Similarly, of 92 cases of gastric cancer during pregnancy reviewed by Jaspers and coworkers [63], nearly all tumors were found in advanced stages, 82% were poorly differentiated, and only 51% were resectable at the time of diagnosis.

In the series by Maeta and coworkers [59], the pregnancy-associated gastric cancer patients had an increased incidence of poorly differentiated adenocarcinoma with scirrhus growth pattern, when compared with age-matched nonpregnant gastric cancer patients. Pregnancy-associated patients had a high incidence of far-advanced stage IV cancer (50%), and the incidence of peritoneal metastasis (42.2%) was significantly higher in the pregnancy-associated cases than in young women with non–pregnancy-associated gastric cancer. Four of the 14 pregnancy-associated cases were detected as early gastric cancer. Of the 14 pregnancy-associated cases, 7 patients who underwent curative surgery (stages I–III) were still alive at last follow-up, whereas all 7 patients with stage IV cancer died of peritoneal metastasis within 1 postoperative year. Early detection of gastric cancer with subsequent curative surgery is the best way to obtain good survival for young pregnant women.

Fetal survival in gastric cancer during pregnancy has been favorable, with 72% survival in Jasper's and coworkers review [63]. For pregnancies greater than 30 weeks, fetal survival was 88% to 100% and only two babies were growth retarded. It is recommended that the decision whether to continue pregnancy can be based on the viability of the baby and the urgency of treatment planned for the patient.

## Pancreatic tumors during pregnancy

### Pancreatic adenocarcinoma

#### Incidence
Pancreatic adenocarcinoma is the fifth leading cause of cancer death among women [72]. It develops infrequently before age 40 years and it has been rare during pregnancy [73]. As of 1997, there had been four reported cases of pancreatic adenocarcinoma during pregnancy [74].

#### Risk factors
A significant portion of patients with pancreatic cancer have a family history of the disease [75]. The genetic factors involved are not yet understood; however, families who have trypsinogen inactivator mutations develop chronic calcific pancreatitis associated with a high incidence of pancreatic cancer [76]. The environmental factors leading to the development of pancreatic cancer have not been clearly defined, although tobacco seems to be a risk factor in some studies [75].

#### Presentation
Pancreatic adenocarcinoma often presents with painless jaundice. The development of jaundice during pregnancy can result from several relatively common disorders, including viral hepatitis, intrahepatic cholestasis of pregnancy, preeclampsia, common bile duct stones, and fatty infiltration of the liver. In most cases, history, physical examination, laboratory tests, and abdominal ultrasound differentiate between hemolysis, hepatocellular, and obstructive disorders with 80% accuracy [77].

#### Diagnosis
Jaundice caused by a pancreatic mass may be suggested by ultrasound detection of dilated bile ducts. Endoscopic retrograde cholangiopancreatography or MR cholangiopancreatography can differentiate between common duct stone,

ampullary neoplasm, bile duct neoplasm, and pancreatic neoplasm. The performance of endoscopic retrograde cholangiopancreatography involves the possible hazard of radiation to the fetus and should be avoided, if possible, before 17 weeks' gestation [78]. Shielding minimizes fetal exposure to radiation. Endoscopic retrograde cholangiopancreatography allows definitive diagnosis; treatment, such as extraction of common bile duct stones or stent placement for palliation of jaundice; and biopsy of ampullary lesions.

Endoscopic ultrasound is a useful method to evaluate the pancreas and does not entail the radiation exposure of endoscopic retrograde cholangiopancreatography [79]. The risks to the fetus should be similar to the risks of upper gastrointestinal endoscopy and some investigators recommend endoscopic ultrasound as a preferred method to evaluate for common bile duct stones during pregnancy [80]. Endoscopic ultrasound also allows biopsy of a pancreatic mass [81].

*Therapy*

*Surgery.* Pancreaticoduodenectomy is the only means for achieving long-term survival for pancreatic adenocarcinoma. Blackbourne and coworkers [74] reported a case of pancreatic adenocarcinoma during pregnancy diagnosed at 17 weeks' gestation. The patient underwent a pylorus-preserving pancreaticoduodenectomy with a choledochojejunostomy, pancreaticojejunostomy, and a duodenojejunostomy. Three months postoperatively, the fetus was developing normally. Simchuk and coworkers [82] diagnosed an unresectable pancreatic adenocarcinoma during pregnancy in a patient who was treated with palliative choledochoduodenostomy and feeding jejunostomy. A healthy baby was delivered by cesarean section at 28 weeks' gestation, whereas the patient died 3 months after surgery. Gamberdella [83] reported a case of unresectable pancreatic carcinoma diagnosed at approximately 24 weeks' gestation, palliated with a decompressing cholecystostomy. At 32 weeks' gestation, healthy twins were delivered by cesarean section and the patient died of metastatic adenocarcinoma of the pancreas 3 months postpartum.

*Chemotherapy.* Multiple adjuvant treatments have been tested for pancreatic carcinoma, most with minimal, if any, effect [84]. Chemotherapy for pancreatic adenocarcinoma using 5-fluorouracil or gemcitabine is palliative and efficacy in the adjuvant setting has not been proved [84,85]. One should be cautious in the use of these drugs, particularly early in pregnancy.

*Prognosis*

Pancreatic adenocarcinoma remains one of the most difficult cancers to treat because it tends to present late and surgical resection is possible in the minority of patients. Only 15% to 20% of patients have resectable disease at presentation with 10% to 20% of resected patients surviving 5 years; however, most of these patients experience late recurrence and ultimately die of the disease [85,86].

## Neuroendocrine tumors

### Incidence

Neuroendocrine tumors of the pancreas are relatively rare, with different subtypes, each occurring at a rate of 1 per million or so in the general population [87]. Islet cell neuroendocrine tumors are the pancreatic neoplasms most frequently diagnosed during pregnancy, with insulinomas being the most common subtype. There are 20 reported cases of insulinoma during pregnancy [88].

### Risk factors

Islet cell tumors are both sporadic and familial, the familial ones being associated with multiple endocrine neoplasia I syndrome [89]. Families with multiple endocrine neoplasia I generally have tumors of the pituitary gland, parathyroid glands, and pancreas, but not all patients have the triad of tumors [90]. In a review of 224 patients with insulinoma, 7.6% were associated with multiple endocrine neoplasia I [91].

### Presentation

The symptoms of insulinoma typically occur with exercise or fasting and include neuroglycopenic symptoms, such as confusion, personality changes, dizziness, weakness, loss of consciousness, and blurred vision. The patient may also experience autonomic symptoms, such as diaphoresis, tremulousness, palpitations, and shortness of breath [92]. Symptoms of central nervous system dysfunction can occur and include seizures, coma, and permanent brain damage [93]. Whipple's triad is used to diagnose a hypoglycemic episode and includes the presence of neuroglycopenic or autonomic symptoms, low plasma glucose at the time of symptoms, and relief of all symptoms with correction of hypoglycemia. Normal pregnancy may produce symptoms similar to those of hypoglycemia, delaying the diagnosis. Fifteen of the 20 pregnant patients who have been described with insulinoma [88] had the onset of symptoms by 16 weeks of gestation. Only one patient had symptoms develop in the third trimester, the only case of metastatic malignant insulinoma during pregnancy reported [88,94]. Later in pregnancy, the normal decrease in insulin sensitivity can create a hyperglycemic state [95]. Patients with insulinoma have a decrease in their symptoms later in pregnancy, and conservative management is suitable [88].

### Diagnosis

The laboratory findings suggestive of insulinoma include a serum insulin level of 10 µU/L or more with plasma glucose levels less than 45 mg/dL [88]. The diagnosis is confirmed with a prolonged, supervised fast, during which serum levels of glucose, insulin, and C-peptide are analyzed [96]. Ultrasound, CT, and MRI have limited sensitivities for preoperative localization of the tumor [97]. Endoscopic ultrasonography may be the most sensitive method for localizing pancreatic islet cell tumors preoperatively [98].

*Therapy*

Because less than 10% of insulinomas are malignant, treatment during pregnancy is the same as in the nonpregnant patient and is directed at controlling hypoglycemic symptoms [91]. The gravid patient with insulinoma may be managed with frequent dietary intake until after delivery. In Takacs' and coworkers series [88], the 14 patients who had symptoms in the first 16 weeks of gestation were treated conservatively and all had resolution of symptoms during the later trimesters. In no case did the disease progress such that the tumor could not be removed or had become metastatic. If diet alone is not sufficient, the patient may be treated with glucagon [88].

Immediate surgery may be necessary for the patient whose disease is worsening significantly during pregnancy. At least 10 cases of surgery for various pancreatic tumors during pregnancy have been reported [74,99,100]. Eight of these operations were uncomplicated and resulted in a term birth; one resulted in delivery at 32 weeks, 1 day after surgery; and one resulted in premature delivery with complications leading to fetal death [100]. The most common surgery was a distal pancreatectomy followed by three pancreaticoduodenectomies. For insulinoma, enucleation of the tumor can sometimes be accomplished [88].

*Prognosis*

The prognosis for insulinoma during pregnancy is generally good for both mother and child as long as prolonged and severe hypoglycemia is avoided [88]. Definitive surgery for neuroendocrine pancreatic tumors presenting during pregnancy can be performed with a good maternal and fetal outcome [100].

**Hepatocellular carcinoma during pregnancy**

*Incidence*

Hepatocellular carcinoma (HCC) seems to be rare during pregnancy in the United States; most reported cases have occurred in Asia and Africa. By 1995 there were approximately 30 reported cases of HCC during pregnancy [101], whereas a more recent review of liver masses in pregnancy reported three additional cases of HCC [102].

*Risk factors*

Risk factors for HCC include chronic hepatitis B, chronic hepatitis C, and cirrhosis from other causes [103]. Aflatoxin in the diet may also be a risk factor for HCC [104]. In 1995, Lau and coworkers [101] reported five cases of HCC during pregnancy and reviewed case reports of 23 additional cases. Among the 25 patients with known racial origin, 8 were Chinese and 6 were Nigerian. Seventeen of these patients had known hepatitis B surface antigen status, with 7 negative and 10 positive patients. Underlying cirrhosis was documented in 10 patients, with 6 cirrhotics being hepatitis B carriers.

*Presentation*

Patients with HCC in pregnancy can present in many ways. Hepatomegaly may be detected on antenatal checkup, although most subjects with hepatomegaly do not have HCC. HCC can present with jaundice, abdominal pain, or very dramatically with shock from liver rupture. In the series by Lau and coworkers [101], four ruptured HCC were identified. Individuals at high risk for HCC may be diagnosed during screening with alpha fetoprotein and liver ultrasound, which are recommended every 6 months in at-risk patients.

*Diagnosis*

Serum alpha fetoprotein levels and liver ultrasound are the main screening tools for detecting HCC in asymptomatic individuals at risk and are used as diagnostic tests in those suspected to have HCC. Because alpha fetoprotein screening of pregnant women is also used for detection of fetal malformations, HCC has sometimes been identified [105,106]. A serum alpha fetoprotein level of greater than 1000 ng/mL, along with a liver mass by ultrasound, is considered diagnostic of HCC. In Lau's series [101], serum alpha fetoprotein levels at presentation were known in 18 cases. Four of the patients had normal alpha fetoprotein levels, 10 patients had levels >400 ng/mL, and the remaining 4 cases had levels between 78 and 270 ng/mL.

*Therapy*

Segmental liver resection is potentially curative in patients with HCC. It is unclear if liver resection is more effective than liver transplantation, although transplantation is generally preferred in subjects with HCC and underlying cirrhosis [107,108]. There is an experience with liver transplantation in the peripartum period for benign diseases, but only after delivery of the fetus [109]. It may be reasonable to attempt resection of HCC early in pregnancy and consider liver transplantation after delivery, although there are not enough cases reported to make firm recommendations. Ablative techniques, such as ethanol injection, radiofrequency ablation, and chemoembolization, are available for treatment of HCC [110]. These techniques are not believed to be curative, but could potentially be used to control disease until more definitive therapy can be provided after delivery. Data for these techniques during pregnancy are lacking.

*Prognosis*

The prognosis for patients with HCC is better for those with smaller tumors. Patients who undergo resection of a tumor less than 1 cm in size have a cure rate that can exceed 80%, whereas those with tumors greater than 5 cm have a cure rate with resection less than 25% [111,112].

As is the case for other gastrointestinal malignancies, pregnancy probably leads to a delay in diagnosis. In the series by Lau and coworkers [101], death occurred rapidly in most cases, with only two patients surviving up to 1 year from diagnosis. Live infants were delivered in about half of the cases (57%).

## Summary

In pregnant patients, colorectal, gastric, pancreatic, and hepatic carcinomas often present as advanced tumors with resulting poor maternal outcomes. Atypical symptoms during pregnancy warrant endoscopic and ultrasound diagnostic testing. When these cancers are diagnosed during the first half of pregnancy, cancer surgery should be promptly performed, without disturbing the pregnancy when possible. With diagnosis later in pregnancy, consideration should be given to delaying treatment until the infant is viable, proceeding with radical surgery after cesarean or induced vaginal delivery. Adjuvant chemotherapy, given in consultation with an oncologist, can be used in the second and third trimesters, but is associated with an increased incidence of prematurity and low-birth-weight infants. Despite this approach, maternal outcomes are poor. Infant survival, however, is favorable.

## References

[1] Jemal A, Thomas A, Murray T, et al. Cancer statistics, 2002. CA Cancer J Clin 2002;52:23–47.
[2] Cappell MS, Goldberg ES. The relationship between the clinical presentation and spread of colon cancer in 315 consecutive patients: a significant trend of earlier cancer detection from 1982 through 1988 at a university hospital. J Clin Gastroenterol 1992;14:227–35.
[3] Isbister WH, Fraser J. Large-bowel cancer in the young: a national survival study. Dis Colon Rectum 1990;33:363–6.
[4] Bernstein MA, Madoff RD, Caushaj PF. Colon and rectal cancer in pregnancy. Dis Colon Rectum 1993;36:172–8.
[5] Woods JB, Martin Jr JN, Ingram FH, et al. Pregnancy complicated by carcinoma of the colon above the rectum. Am J Perinatol 1992;9:102–10.
[6] Cappell MS. Colon cancer during pregnancy. Gastroenterol Clin North Am 2003;32:341–83.
[7] Jarvinen HJ. Epidemiology of familial adenomatous polyposis in Finland: impact of family screening on the colorectal cancer rate and survival. Gut 1992;33:357–60.
[8] Burt RW. Familial risk and colorectal cancer. Gastroenterol Clin North Am 1996;25:793–803.
[9] Itzkowitz SH. Inflammatory bowel disease and cancer. Gastroenterol Clin North Am 1997;26: 129–39.
[10] Girard RM, Lamarche J, Baillot R. Carcinoma of the colon associated with pregnancy: report of a case. Dis Colon Rectum 1981;24:473–5.
[11] Nesbitt JC, Moise KJ, Sawyers JL. Colorectal carcinoma in pregnancy. Arch Surg 1985;120: 636–40.
[12] Winawer S, Fletcher R, Rex D, et al. Colorectal cancer screening and surveillance: clinical guidelines and rationale. Update based on new evidence. Gastroenterology 2003;124:544–60.
[13] Ransohoff DF, Lang CA. Screening for colorectal cancer. N Engl J Med 1991;325:37–41.
[14] Bentley DP. Iron metabolism and anaemia in pregnancy. Clin Haematol 1985;14:613–28.
[15] Shushan A, Stemmer SM, Reubinoff BE, et al. Carcinoma of the colon during pregnancy. Obstet Gynecol Surv 1992;47:222–5.
[16] Brent RL. The effect of embryonic and fetal exposure to x-ray, microwaves, and ultrasound: counseling the pregnant and nonpregnant patient about these risks. Semin Oncol 1989;16: 347–68.
[17] Reece EA, Assimakopoulos E, Zheng XZ, et al. The safety of obstetric ultrasonography: concern for the fetus. Obstet Gynecol 1990;76:139–46.
[18] Nies C, Leppek R, Sitter H, et al. Prospective evaluation of different diagnostic techniques for

the detection of liver metastases at the time of primary resection of colorectal carcinoma. Eur J Surg 1996;162:811–6.

[19] Devesa SS, Chow WH. Variation in colorectal cancer incidence in the United States by subsite of origin. Cancer 1993;71:3819–26.

[20] Schoenfeld P, Cash B, Flood A, et al. Colonoscopic screening of average-risk women for colorectal neoplasia. N Engl J Med 2005;352:2061–8.

[21] Cappell MS. The fetal safety and clinical efficacy of gastrointestinal endoscopy during pregnancy. Gastroenterol Clin North Am 2003;32:123–79.

[22] Cappell MS, Colon VJ, Sidhom OA. A study at 10 medical centers of the safety and efficacy of 48 flexible sigmoidoscopies and 8 colonoscopies during pregnancy with follow-up of fetal outcome and with comparison to control groups. Dig Dis Sci 1996;41:2353–61.

[23] Cappell MS, Fiest TC. A multicenter, multiyear, case-controlled study of the risk of colonic polyps in patients with gastric polyps. Are gastric adenomas a new indication for surveillance colonoscopy? J Clin Gastroenterol 1995;21:198–202.

[24] Koness RJ, King TC, Schechter S, et al. Synchronous colon carcinomas: molecular-genetic evidence for multicentricity. Ann Surg Oncol 1996;3:136–43.

[25] Zauber AG, Winawer SJ. Initial management and follow-up surveillance of patients with colorectal adenomas. Gastroenterol Clin North Am 1997;26:85–101.

[26] Bashir RM, Montgomery EA, Gupta PK, et al. Massive gastrointestinal hemorrhage during pregnancy caused by ectopic decidua of the terminal ileum and colon. Am J Gastroenterol 1995;90:1325–7.

[27] Gonsoulin W, Mason B, Carpenter Jr RJ. Colon cancer in pregnancy with elevated maternal serum alpha-fetoprotein level at presentation. Am J Obstet Gynecol 1990;163(4 Pt 1): 1172–3.

[28] Rojansky N, Shushan A, Livni N, et al. Pregnancy associated with colon carcinoma overexpressing p53. Gynecol Oncol 1997;64:516–20.

[29] Morrison JC, Wiser WL, Rosser SI, et al. Metabolites of meperidine related to fetal depression. Am J Obstet Gynecol 1973;115:1132–7.

[30] Abboud TK, Zhu J, Richardson M, et al. Intravenous propofol vs thiamylal-isoflurane for caesarean section, comparative maternal and neonatal effects. Acta Anaesthesiol Scand 1995;39:205–9.

[31] Cheng YJ, Wang YP, Fan SZ, et al. Intravenous infusion of low dose propofol for conscious sedation in cesarean section before spinal anesthesia. Acta Anaesthesiol Sin 1997;35:79–84.

[32] Fisher ER, Sass R, Palekar A, et al. Dukes' classification revisited. Findings from the National Surgical Adjuvant Breast and Bowel Projects (Protocol R-01). Cancer 1989;64:2354–60.

[33] Malangoni MA. Gastrointestinal surgery and pregnancy. Gastroenterol Clin North Am 2003;32:181–200.

[34] Walsh C, Fazio VW. Cancer of the colon, rectum, and anus during pregnancy: the surgeon's perspective. Gastroenterol Clin North Am 1998;27:257–67.

[35] Arbman G, Nilsson E, Storgren-Fordell V, et al. A short diagnostic delay is more important for rectal cancer than for colonic cancer. Eur J Surg 1996;162:899–904.

[36] Skilling JS. Colorectal cancer complicating pregnancy. Obstet Gynecol Clin North Am 1998;25:417–21.

[37] Medich DS, Fazio VW. Hemorrhoids, anal fissure, and carcinoma of the colon, rectum, and anus during pregnancy. Surg Clin North Am 1995;75:77–88.

[38] Diaz-Rubio E. New chemotherapeutic advances in pancreatic, colorectal, and gastric cancers. Oncologist 2004;9:282–94.

[39] Moertel CG, Fleming TR, Macdonald JS, et al. Levamisole and fluorouracil for adjuvant therapy of resected colon carcinoma. N Engl J Med 1990;322:352–8.

[40] Aviles A, Diaz-Maqueo JC, Talavera A, et al. Growth and development of children of mothers treated with chemotherapy during pregnancy: current status of 43 children. Am J Hematol 1991;36:243–8.

[41] Fleshman JW, Myerson RJ. Adjuvant radiation therapy for adenocarcinoma of the rectum. Surg Clin North Am 1997;77:15–25.

[42] Kido A, Mori M, Adachi Y, et al. Immunohistochemical expression of beta-human chorionic gonadotropin in colorectal carcinoma. Surg Today 1996;26:966–70.

[43] Krause H, Watt A. Positive pregnancy test in a patient with colorectal carcinoma. Aust N Z J Obstet Gynaecol 2003;43:241–2.

[44] Braunstein GD, Vaitukaitis JL, Carbone PP, et al. Ectopic production of human chorionic gonadotrophin by neoplasms. Ann Intern Med 1973;78:39–45.

[45] Campo E, Palacin A, Benasco C, et al. Human chorionic gonadotropin in colorectal carcinoma: an immunohistochemical study. Cancer 1987;59:1611–6.

[46] Skinner JM, Whitehead R. Tumor-associated antigens in polyps and carcinoma of the human large bowel. Cancer 1981;47:1241–5.

[47] Buckley CH, Fox H. An immunohistochemical study of the significance of HCG secretion by large bowel adenocarcinomata. J Clin Pathol 1979;32:368–72.

[48] Herrera-Ornelas L, Natarajan N, Tsukada Y, et al. Adenocarcinoma of the colon masquerading as primary ovarian neoplasia: an analysis of ten cases. Dis Colon Rectum 1983;26: 377–80.

[49] Mason III MH, Kovalcik PJ. Ovarian metastases from colon carcinoma. J Surg Oncol 1981;17:33–8.

[50] Pitluk H, Poticha SM. Carcinoma of the colon and rectum in patients less than 40 years of age. Surg Gynecol Obstet 1983;157:335–7.

[51] Recalde M, Holyoke ED, Elias EG. Carcinoma of the colon, rectum, and anal canal in young patients. Surg Gynecol Obstet 1974;139:909–13.

[52] Tsukamoto N, Uchino H, Matsukuma K, et al. Carcinoma of the colon presenting as bilateral ovarian tumors during pregnancy. Gynecol Oncol 1986;24:386–91.

[53] Matsuyama T, Tsukamoto N, Matsukuma K, et al. Malignant ovarian tumors associated with pregnancy: report of six cases. Int J Gynaecol Obstet 1989;28:61–6.

[54] Rothman LA, Cohen CJ, Astarloa J. Placental and fetal involvement by maternal malignancy: a report of rectal carcinoma and review of the literature. Am J Obstet Gynecol 1973;116: 1023–34.

[55] Kort B, Katz VL, Watson WJ. The effect of nonobstetric operation during pregnancy. Surg Gynecol Obstet 1993;177:371–6.

[56] Hill JA, Kassam SH, Talledo OE. Colonic cancer in pregnancy. South Med J 1984;77:375–8.

[57] Mitsudomi T, Matsusaka T, Wakasugi K, et al. A clinicopathological study of gastric cancer with special reference to age of the patients: an analysis of 1,630 cases. World J Surg 1989;13:225–30 [discussion: 221–30].

[58] Okamoto T, Makino M, Kawasumi H, et al. Comparative study of gastric cancer in young and aged patients. Eur Surg Res 1988;20:149–55.

[59] Maeta M, Yamashiro H, Oka A, et al. Gastric cancer in the young, with special reference to 14 pregnancy-associated cases: analysis based on 2,325 consecutive cases of gastric cancer. J Surg Oncol 1995;58:191–5.

[60] Parkin DM, Pisani P, Ferlay J. Estimates of the worldwide incidence of eighteen major cancers in 1985. Int J Cancer 1993;54:594–606.

[61] Bloss RS, Miller TA, Copeland III EM. Carcinoma of the stomach in the young adult. Surg Gynecol Obstet 1980;150:883–6.

[62] Kurabayashi T, Isii K, Suzuki M, et al. Advanced gastric cancer and a concomitant pregnancy associated with disseminated intravascular coagulation. Am J Perinatol 2004;21:295–8.

[63] Jaspers VK, Gillessen A, Quakernack K. Gastric cancer in pregnancy: do pregnancy, age or female sex alter the prognosis? Case reports and review. Eur J Obstet Gynecol Reprod Biol 1999;87:13–22.

[64] Ueo H, Matsuoka H, Tamura S, et al. Prognosis in gastric cancer associated with pregnancy. World J Surg 1991;15:293–7 [discussion: 298].

[65] Kelley JR, Duggan JM. Gastric cancer epidemiology and risk factors. J Clin Epidemiol 2003;56:1–9.

[66] Janulaityte-Gunther D, Kupcinskas L, Pavilonis A, et al. *Helicobacter pylori* antibodies and gastric cancer: a gender-related difference. FEMS Immunol Med Microbiol 2005;44:191–5.

[67] Eliakim R, Abulafia O, Sherer DM. Hyperemesis gravidarum: a current review. Am J Perinatol 2000;17:207–18.

[68] Fazeny B, Marosi C. Gastric cancer as an essential differential diagnosis of minor epigastric discomfort during pregnancy. Acta Obstet Gynecol Scand 1998;77:469–71.

[69] Lordick F, Siewert JR. Recent advances in multimodal treatment for gastric cancer: a review. Gastric Cancer 2005;8:78–85.

[70] Moehler M, Schimanski CC, Gockel I, et al. (Neo)adjuvant strategies of advanced gastric carcinoma: time for a change? Dig Dis 2004;22:345–50.

[71] Dupont Jr JB, Lee JR, Burton GR, et al. Adenocarcinoma of the stomach: review of 1,497 cases. Cancer 1978;41:941–7.

[72] Boring CC, Squires TS, Tong T, et al. Cancer statistics, 1994. CA Cancer J Clin 1994;44:7–26.

[73] Donegan WL. Cancer and pregnancy. CA Cancer J Clin 1983;33:194–214.

[74] Blackbourne LH, Jones RS, Catalano CJ, et al. Pancreatic adenocarcinoma in the pregnant patient: case report and review of the literature. Cancer 1997;79:1776–9.

[75] James TA, Sheldon DG, Rajput A, et al. Risk factors associated with earlier age of onset in familial pancreatic carcinoma. Cancer 2004;101:2722–6.

[76] Howes N, Greenhalf W, Stocken DD, et al. Cationic trypsinogen mutations and pancreatitis. Gastroenterol Clin North Am 2004;33:767–87.

[77] Schenker S, Balint J, Schiff L. Differential diagnosis of jaundice: report of a prospective study of 61 proved cases. Am J Dig Dis 1962;7:449–63.

[78] Tham TC, Vandervoort J, Wong RC, et al. Safety of ERCP during pregnancy. Am J Gastroenterol 2003;98:308–11.

[79] Snady H. Endoscopic ultrasonography in benign pancreatic disease. Surg Clin North Am 2001;81:329–44.

[80] Norton SA, Alderson D. Prospective comparison of endoscopic ultrasonography and endoscopic retrograde cholangiopancreatography in the detection of bile duct stones. Br J Surg 1997;84:1366–9.

[81] Chang KJ, Nguyen P, Erickson RA, et al. The clinical utility of endoscopic ultrasound-guided fine-needle aspiration in the diagnosis and staging of pancreatic carcinoma. Gastrointest Endosc 1997;45:387–93.

[82] Simchuk III EJ, Welch JP, Orlando III R. Antepartum diagnosis of pancreatic carcinoma: a case report. Conn Med 1995;59:259–62.

[83] Gamberdella FR. Pancreatic carcinoma in pregnancy: a case report. Am J Obstet Gynecol 1984;149:15–7.

[84] Van Cutsem E, Aerts R, Haustermans K, et al. Systemic treatment of pancreatic cancer. Eur J Gastroenterol Hepatol 2004;16:265–74.

[85] Brennan MF. Adjuvant therapy following resection for pancreatic adenocarcinoma. Surg Oncol Clin N Am 2004;13:555–66.

[86] Li D, Xie K, Wolff R, et al. Pancreatic cancer. Lancet 2004;363:1049–57.

[87] Eriksson B, Oberg K, Skogseid B. Neuroendocrine pancreatic tumors: clinical findings in a prospective study of 84 patients. Acta Oncol 1989;28:373–7.

[88] Takacs CA, Krivak TC, Napolitano PG. Insulinoma in pregnancy: a case report and review of the literature. Obstet Gynecol Surv 2002;57:229–35.

[89] Jensen RT. Pancreatic endocrine tumors: recent advances. Ann Oncol 1999;10(Suppl 4): 170–6.

[90] Marx S, Spiegel AM, Skarulis MC, et al. Multiple endocrine neoplasia type 1: clinical and genetic topics. Ann Intern Med 1998;129:484–94.

[91] Service FJ, McMahon MM, O'Brien PC, et al. Functioning insulinoma: incidence, recurrence, and long-term survival of patients: a 60-year study. Mayo Clin Proc 1991;66:711–9.

[92] Dizon AM, Kowalyk S, Hoogwerf BJ. Neuroglycopenic and other symptoms in patients with insulinomas. Am J Med 1999;106:307–10.

[93] Grant CS. Insulinoma. Surg Oncol Clin N Am 1998;7:819–44.

[94] Friedman E, Moses B, Engelberg S, et al. Malignant insulinoma with hepatic failure complicating pregnancy. South Med J 1988;81:86–8.

[95]  Ryan EA, Enns L. Role of gestational hormones in the induction of insulin resistance. J Clin Endocrinol Metab 1988;67:341–7.

[96]  Service FJ. Hypoglycemic disorders. N Engl J Med 1995;332:1144–52.

[97]  Smythe II AR, McFarland KF, Yousufuddin M, et al. Multiple endocrine adenomatosis type I in pregnancy. Am J Obstet Gynecol 1990;163:1037–8 [discussion 1038–9].

[98]  McLean AM, Fairclough PD. Endoscopic ultrasound in the localisation of pancreatic islet cell tumours. Best Pract Res Clin Endocrinol Metab 2005;19:177–93.

[99]  Ganepola GA, Gritsman AY, Asimakopulos N, et al. Are pancreatic tumors hormone dependent? A case report of unusual, rapidly growing pancreatic tumor during pregnancy, its possible relationship to female sex hormones, and review of the literature. Am Surg 1999;65: 105–11.

[100] Sciscione AC, Villeneuve JB, Pitt HA, et al. Surgery for pancreatic tumors during pregnancy: a case report and review of the literature. Am J Perinatol 1996;13:21–5.

[101] Lau WY, Leung WT, Ho S, et al. Hepatocellular carcinoma during pregnancy and its comparison with other pregnancy-associated malignancies. Cancer 1995;75:2669–76.

[102] Cobey FC, Salem RR. A review of liver masses in pregnancy and a proposed algorithm for their diagnosis and management. Am J Surg 2004;187:181–91.

[103] Zhang JY, Dai M, Wang X, et al. A case-control study of hepatitis B and C virus infection as risk factors for hepatocellular carcinoma in Henan, China. Int J Epidemiol 1998;27:574–8.

[104] Cha C, Dematteo RP. Molecular mechanisms in hepatocellular carcinoma development. Best Pract Res Clin Gastroenterol 2005;19:25–37.

[105] Entezami M, Becker R, Ebert A, et al. Hepatocellular carcinoma as a rare cause of an excessive increase in alpha-fetoprotein during pregnancy. Gynecol Oncol 1996;62:405–7.

[106] Jeng LB, Lee WC, Wang CC, et al. Hepatocellular carcinoma in a pregnant woman detected by routine screening of maternal alpha-fetoprotein. Am J Obstet Gynecol 1995;172(1 Pt 1): 219–20.

[107] Philosophe B, Greig PD, Hemming AW, et al. Surgical management of hepatocellular carcinoma: resection or transplantation? J Gastrointest Surg 1998;2:21–7.

[108] Pierie JP, Muzikansky A, Tanabe KK, et al. The outcome of surgical resection versus assignment to the liver transplant waiting list for hepatocellular carcinoma. Ann Surg Oncol 2005;12(7):552–60.

[109] Shames BD, Fernandez LA, Sollinger HW, et al. Liver transplantation for HELLP syndrome. Liver Transpl 2005;11:224–8.

[110] Jansen MC, van Hillegersberg R, Chamuleau RA, et al. Outcome of regional and local ablative therapies for hepatocellular carcinoma: a collective review. Eur J Surg Oncol 2005;31:331–47.

[111] Poon RT, Fan ST, Lo CM, et al. Long-term prognosis after resection of hepatocellular carcinoma associated with hepatitis B-related cirrhosis. J Clin Oncol 2000;18:1094–101.

[112] Shimozawa N, Hanazaki K. Long-term prognosis after hepatic resection for small hepatocellular carcinoma. J Am Coll Surg 2004;198:356–65.

ELSEVIER
SAUNDERS

Obstet Gynecol Clin N Am
32 (2005) 661–684

OBSTETRICS AND
GYNECOLOGY
CLINICS
OF NORTH AMERICA

# Choriocarcinoma and Gestational Trophoblastic Disease

## Harriet O. Smith, MD[a],*, Ernest Kohorn, MD[b], Laurence A. Cole, PhD[a]

[a]*University of New Mexico Health Sciences Center, Division of Gynecologic Oncology, Department of Obstetrics and Gynecology, 2211 Lomas Boulevard, NE, Albuquerque, NM 87131-5286, USA*
[b]*Department of Gynecology, Yale University School of Medicine, 333 Cedar Street, New Haven, CT 06510, USA*

The term gestational trophoblastic disease (GTD) encompasses a unique group of uncommon but interrelated conditions derived from placental trophoblasts that differ in propensity for regression, invasion, metastasis, and recurrence [1]. The World Health Organization divides GTD into the following groups: complete hydatidiform mole (CM), partial mole (PM), choriocarcinoma, placental site trophoblastic tumor (PSTT), miscellaneous trophoblastic tumor (exaggerated placental site, placental site nodule or plaque), and unclassified trophoblastic lesions [2]. For the purposes of discussion and treatment, gestational trophoblastic disease is the appropriate collective name for hydatidiform mole (complete, partial, invasive with resolution of human chorionic gonadotropin [hCG]), whereas the term gestational trophoblastic neoplasia (GTN) is reserved for cases with persistent hCG titer elevation after evacuation of hydatidiform mole, metastatic disease, or choriocarcinoma [3,4].

## Pathology of molar subtypes

Both partial and complete molar pregnancies are characterized by the presence of hydropic villi. The classical appearance of complete moles is large edematous

---

\* Corresponding author.
*E-mail address:* Hsmith@salud.unm.edu (H.O. Smith).

0889-8545/05/$ – see front matter © 2005 Elsevier Inc. All rights reserved.
doi:10.1016/j.ogc.2005.08.001 *obgyn.theclinics.com*

clusters of vesicles 0.5 to 2 cm in size (Fig. 1), with varying amounts of hemorrhage and necrosis. When compared with historic controls, fewer patients today present with the traditional more aggressive symptoms of complete hydatidiform mole (excessive uterine size, anemia, preeclampsia, hyperthyroidism, or hyperemesis), although the rate of postmolar GTN has not appreciably declined [5]. Because of the widespread use of obstetric ultrasound, molar pregnancies are more likely to be diagnosed at 8.5–9.5 weeks instead of 16–18 weeks estimated gestational age (EGA), which may account for the change in clinical presentation [5,6]. The structural resolution by ultrasound is 3 mm; therefore, hydatidiform mole is unlikely to be detected on ultrasound before 6-8 weeks EGA. Kajii and colleagues [7–9] demonstrated the androgenetic origin of complete or classic hydatidiform mole. In CM, the nuclear DNA is exclusively of paternal origin. The majority are 46XX [10], and arise from fertilization of an empty pronucleus by a haploid sperm that undergoes duplication, a condition referred to as diandric diploidy. Although most of the remainder are 46XY, which arise from the fertilization of an empty egg by two sperm and are termed diandric dispermy [6,9,11], other karyotypic types have been reported, including tetraploidy [12]. For CM, the risk for GTN following evacuation is approximately 15%–20%. Risk is influenced by the initial hCG titer (serum hCG over 100,000 mIU/mL,

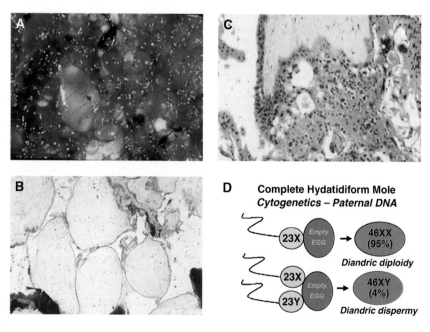

Fig. 1. Complete hydatidiform mole (CM). (*A*) Enlarged and edematous grape-like vesicles 0.5 to 2 cm in size. Molar villi obtained on suction dilation and evacuation may be collapsed and obscured by accompanying blood, but can be reconstituted in hypotonic saline. (*B*) Microscopically, CM villi have large acellular central cisterna. A fetus, fetal parts, or fetal red blood cells are absent. (*C*) Trophoblastic proliferation is circumferential, completely surrounding the villus, and varying degrees of cellular atypia are present. (*D*) Most common cytogenetics of complete mole.

the rate of decline of hCG [13], the presence of large theca lutein cysts, and the method of evacuation [6,13].

Like CM, partial moles (PM) have less abundant hydropic villi that are large and edematous with at least focal central cisterns, as well as smaller villi that display stromal fibrosis (Fig. 2). Typically, the karyotype of PM is triploidy (69 chromosomes), which result from fertilization of an oocyte by either a duplicated spermatozoa or two spermatozoa, termed monogynic diandric triploidy. Of these, 70% are 69, XXY; 27% are 69, XXX; and 3% are 69, XYY [14]. These are distinguished cytogenetically from triploid conceptuses, which have a diploid set of maternal DNA and a haploid set of paternal DNA, or digenic tripoidy [15–17]. Although complete mole does not usually present a diagnostic dilemma, it can be difficult or impossible to distinguish PM from a hydropic abortus using light microscopy alone, and ploidy studies may be useful [18–21]. In contrast to PM pregnancies, missed abortions are typically triploid with two maternal and one paternal haploid, and are termed digenic tripoidy. Because PM can be clinically and cytologically confused with missed abortion, the risk of postmolar recurrence in these cases has received a fair amount of consideration. Following evacuation of partial moles (PM), the risk of GTN development is low. Series in

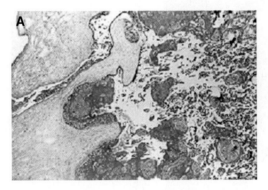

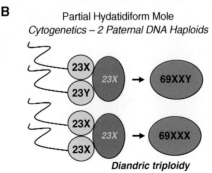

**B** Partial Hydatidiform Mole
*Cytogenetics – 2 Paternal DNA Haploids*

*Diandric triploidy*

Fig. 2. Partial hydatidiform mole (PM). (*A*) Normal and hydropic villi. Usually, villi contain fetal vessels and fetal red blood cells. (*B*) Most commonly PMs arise from the fertilization of a haploid egg by two sperm.

the United States indicate the rate of recurrence is 2%–4%, and 1.8% in the largest series of partial moles (2627 cases) reported to date [22]. Patients who have PM rarely develop metastatic disease [23,24] or transform into choriocarcinoma [22]. Follow-up, using hCG titers, is recommended for all patients who have tripoidy pregnancies until they normalize. However, from the standpoint of GTN prevention, there is no proven benefit of cytogenetics on patients who have either partial mole or missed abortion, to ensure surveillance.

## Choriocarcinoma and placental site trophoblastic tumor

Gestational choriocarcinoma is a relatively rare and highly malignant variant that must be distinguished from non-gestational germ cell tumors [15,25]. Choriocarcinoma can be preceded by any gestational event: 50% arise after hydatidiform mole, 25% after spontaneous abortion, 22.5% after a normal pregnancy, and 2.5% following ectopic pregnancy [26]. Usually, but not always, the predisposing pregnancy is the one most temporally related [27]. There is

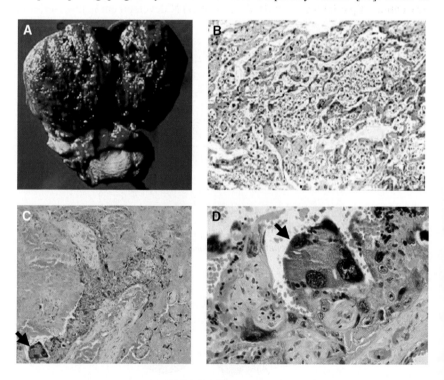

Fig. 3. (A) Choriocarcinoma, characterized by rapid invasive growth with hemorrhage and necrosis. (B) Choriocarcinoma histopathology; clusters and sheets of cytotrophoblasts surrounded by multinucleated syncytiotrophoblasts. (C,D) Choriocarcinoma in-situ; characteristic biphasic pattern of cytotrophoblast and syncytiotrophoblast. Choriocarcinoma is surrounded and arose from otherwise normal appearing villi with projections of tumor cells into the intervillous space.

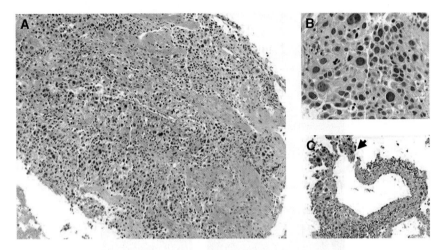

Fig. 4. Placental site trophoblastic tumor (PSTT). Cells strongly resemble intermediate trophoblasts of the implantation sites. (*A*) Low power, characteristic splaying of smooth muscle fascicles by intermediate trophoblastic cells. (*B*) Higher power demonstrating increased mitotic activity and marked pleomorphism. (*C*) Tumor cells can undermine endometrial vein wall, with replacement of vessel wall with fibrinous material (*arrow*).

considerable variation in the rate of choriocarcinoma per pregnancy in different regions of the world. In Europe and North America, choriocarcinoma has been reported in every 30,000–40,000 intrauterine, and 1 in 40 molar pregnancies [25,28–30]. Rates are as high as 1 in every 500–3000 pregnancies in Southeast Asia [31]. These highly vascular neoplasms readily metastasize, most commonly to the lung (60%–75%), the vagina (40%–50%), brain (15%–20%), liver (15%–20%), spleen (10%), and intestines (10%). However, any part of the body can be affected [32–34]. The risk of hemorrhage from biopsy often discourages histological confirmation. Thus, treatment is based upon the number and location of lesions, timing of the antecedent pregnancy, and the hCG titer [13], rather than on histological confirmation. Grossly, the tumor is characterized by hemorrhage and necrosis (Figs. 3–6) and microscopically, by sheets and clusters of

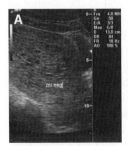
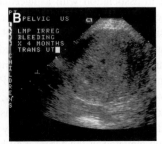
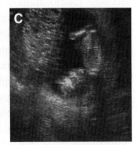

Fig. 5. (*A*) Classic snowstorm appearance of a complete mole. (*B*) Partial mole with degenerating placenta and no fetus. (*C*) intrauterine pregnancy with normal twin and complete hydatidiform mole.

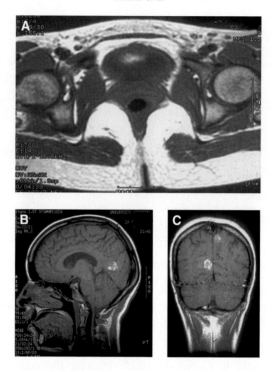

Fig. 6. High-risk GTD. (*A*) Suspicious uterine fundic mass in a patient with rising hCG titers after multiagent chemotherapy including EMA-CO. At hysterectomy, no gross lesion was seen, but under light microscopy a 1-cm lesion, histologically consistent with choriocarcinoma, was found. (*B,C*) The same patient developed two brain lesions, one in the right medial occipital lobe and the second in the left posterior parietal lobe, which were found three months later. Athough this patient had received many different regimens including ifosphamide and bleomycin-cisplatin-based regimens as well as single-agent paclitaxel, she was ultimately salvaged with intrathecal methotrexate, actinomycin D, and etoposide and whole brain irradiation (follow-up 8 years).

cytotrophoblasts and multinucleated syncytiotrophoblastic cells. Except in the rare case of choriocarcinoma with a term pregnancy, villi are absent [26,35,36]. Because choriocarcinoma in association with a placenta and in the absence of metastatic disease is exceedingly rare, there is reluctance on the part of pathologists to make the diagnosis. This can result in treatment delays [35,36].

PSTT, epitheliod trophoblastic tumor, and exaggerated placental site/placental site nodule are rare variants of GTD and have differing risks for GTN. Once considered to be a benign condition, when metastatic, PSTT can be difficult to control even with surgery and aggressive chemotherapy. PSTT arises from neoplastic intermediate trophoblastic cells, and is usually associated with low hCG levels. Human placental lactogen (HPL) may generally be detected by immunohistochemistry, and when elevated in the serum may be used for surveillance. Like choriocarinoma, PSTT may arise following any type of gestational event. The most common presenting symptoms are vaginal bleeding and amenorrhea.

Although the diagnosis can sometimes be made by uterine curettage, the definitive diagnosis is usually made by hysterectomy, which is also the treatment of choice. Most cases are confined to the uterus, but metastasis has been reported in the lung and other sites, and a diligent search for metastatic disease is essential. Compared with other GTN variants, PSTT is less sensitive to chemotherapy. The best responses reported to date have been with the combination regimens EMA-CO (etoposide, actinomycin D, methotrexate, cytoxan, vincristine) or EMA-EP (etoposide, methotrexate, actinomycin D, etoposide, cisplatin) [37–40].

## Initial clinical management

Although the pathology and clinical behavior of CM and PM are different, the initial management of both conditions is basically the same: surgical evacuation by suction curettage, determination of the baseline, and follow-up with hCG titers [1]. Before evacuation of a PM, laminaria may be used to dilate the cervix, but should not be removed until immediately before suction curettage. In addition to diagnosis, ultrasound may be used to ensure complete evacuation and reduce the risk of uterine perforation. Ultrasound has also been used following evacuation to determine if there is residual molar tissue that should be removed, before initiating chemotherapy [41–43]. Other essential studies include a baseline pre-evacuation hCG titer, a preoperative chest radiograph to evaluate for pulmonary metastases or evidence of high-output cardiac failure, and blood type and cross match. Pulmonary complications may occur from trophoblastic deportation, volume overload, hyperthyroidism, and preeclampsia. There is substantial evidence that hCG is a weak thyrotropin (TSH) agonist, and some patients who have GTD express a variant of hCG with increased thyroid-stimulating activity [44–46]. Patients who have high hCG levels (200,000 mIU/ML) may exhibit evidence of acute hyperthyroidism and benefit from $\beta$-blockers perioperatively. Trophoblastic deportation has received emphasis as a cause for respiratory failure; however, high output cardiac failure from severe anemia and excessive hydration is a more common complication. This can usually be prevented by volume management. Pulmonary artery or central venous pressure monitoring can be helpful in patients who have cardiopulmonary insufficiency of uncertain etiology. Patients who are Rh-negative should be treated with anti-D immune globulin. Theca-lutein cysts result from hCG stimulation of the ovaries and may take several months to resolve. Surgical intervention for theca lutein cysts is not indicated except for rupture or torsion.

Following evacuation, patients should be evaluated by serial quantitative serum hCG determinations preoperatively, within 48 hours post evacuation, weekly until values normalize, and then monthly for at least 6 months. Opinions differ about the length of time patients should be followed with monthly hCG titers after normalization of values, and both 6-month and 1-year surveillance have been recommended. There are rare, isolated cases of post molar GTN in patients a year after diagnosis [47]. In one large series of untreated molar pregnancies, the risk of persistent GTN in patients with normalization of hCG (< 5 mIU/mL) was extremely low: 0.2% (2/876, 95% CI 0%–0.8%) [48]. Patients undergoing post evacuation surveillance should consistently use effective contraception to reduce the risk of another pregnancy, which would complicate surveillance. There is some dispute about the influence of oral contraceptive (OC) use on the rate of hCG decline. Some reports indicate an increased risk [49–51], whereas others report no adverse effect [52,53]. Perhaps of greater importance, compared with barrier contraception, OC use has been shown to reduce the risk of conception during post-molar surveillance by 50%, with no increase in persistent GTN [52]. It has also been reported that OC use increases the risk of developing a molar pregnancy [51], but expert opinion holds that this risk is small compared with the benefit of preventing an unwanted pregnancy.

**Staging systems for gestational trophoblastic neoplasia**

In contrast to other gynecologic malignancies, there are four different staging classifications for GTN. These include the Hammond Clinical Classification, the World Health Organization (WHO), the International Federation Gynecology and Obstetrics (FIGO), and the Bagshawe or Charing Cross Risk Fetus Scores system [54]. Of these, the FIGO staging system was the least well known or used in the United States, perhaps because previous FIGO staging grouped high- with low-risk GTN (ie, included vaginal metastases with other metastases that are known to confer a worse prognosis). The 1992 risk factor modifications were radically revised in 2000 (Tables 1,2) to simplify staging, to differentiate high- from low-risk GTN, and to replace the 1992 FIGO risk factor scoring system with the more uniformly accepted system adapted by WHO from Bagshawe. Since then, reports indicate that these proposed changes are accomplishing the primary goal of the staging system, which is to classify untreated patients into distinct prognostic categories so that treatment outcomes can be objectively compared. The new risk factor scoring system eliminated the ABO blood group risk factors, and the risk for liver metastasis was upgraded from 2 to 4.

Table 1
Anatomic FIGO staging system for GTN

| Stage | Indicator |
| --- | --- |
| Stage I | Disease confined to the uterus |
| Stage II | Disease outside of uterus but limited to genital structures |
| Stage III | Disease extends to lungs with or without genital tract involvement |
| Stage IV | All other metastatic sites |

*Adapted from* Kohorn EI. The new FIGO 2000 staging and risk factor scoring system for gestational trophoblastic disease: description and critical assessment. Int J Gynecol Cancer 2001;11(1):73–7.

Table 2
The scoring system for FIGO 2000 staging

| FIGO score | 0 | 1 | 2 | 4 |
|---|---|---|---|---|
| Age | $\leq 40$ years | $>40$ years | — | — |
| Antecedent pregnancy | H. mole | Abortion | Term | |
| Number of months since index pregnancy | $<4$ | 4–6 | 7–12 | $>12$ |
| Pretreatment hCG (mIU/mL) | $<10^3$ | $10^3$–$10^4$ | $>10^4$–$10^5$ | $>10^5$ |
| Largest tumor size including uterus | 3–4 cm | 5 cm | — | — |
| Site(s) of metastasis | — | Spleen, kidney | gastrointestinal tract | Brain, liver |
| Number of metastases | 0 | 1–4 | 4–8 | $>8$ |
| Previously failed chemotherapy | — | — | Single agent | 2 or more agents |

*Adapted from* Kohorn EI. The new FIGO 2000 staging and risk factor scoring system for gestational trophoblastic disease: description and critical assessment. Int J Gynecol Cancer 2001;11(1):73–7.

One of the most significant changes recommended was the inclusion of explicit criteria for the diagnosis of GTN following the evacuation of a hydatidiform mole.

Four values or more of plateau of hCG over at least 3 weeks, drawn on days 1, 7, 14, and 21
A rise of hCG of 10% or more as determined by 3 consecutive values obtained over 2 or more weeks (eg, days 1, 7, and 14)
The presence of choriocarcinoma
Persistence of a positive hCG titer 6 months after evacuation.

The leading trophoblastic centers in Europe and America recommend withholding treatment when hCG titers are below 100 mIU/mL, or even below 200 mIU/mL, in the absence of a clear, upward trend, as this may represent quiescent or inactive gestational trophoblastic disease [55–61].

The radiographic procedures to define metastasis were also standardized. The chest radiograph should be used to count the number of metastases for risk score assessment, although both chest radiograph and CT scan are acceptable to detect metastatic disease. Both ultrasound and CT scan can be used to identify liver metastasis, but a CT scan is preferable. For brain metastases, MRI is preferable to CT scanning, even with 1 cm cuts. In terms of the FIGO risk score system, the intermediate group within WHO has been eliminated, and patients are defined as low risk if the risk score is 6 or less, and high risk if the score is 7 or greater.

When the diagnosis of GTN is suspected, clinical and radiographic assessment of risk is performed. This should include history (most recent antecedent pregnancy and type), physical examination, a complete blood count with differential and platelets, liver and renal function studies, blood type and antibody screen, verification that the positive hCG test is truly indicative of persistent trophoblastic disease and not a false-positive [62,63], chest radiograph, chest CT (and abdominal CT if the chest radiograph is positive), and ultrasonography [1]. GTN usually spreads by the hematogenous route [64] and distant metastases rarely occur in the absence of pulmonary metastases [65]. However, patients with a negative chest radiograph can have occult pulmonary lesions detectable by chest CT in up to 43% of cases. For this reason, a chest CT may be a useful marker to identify patients who require additional evaluation for metastatic lesions [66–68]. On the other hand, micrometastases on chest CT may be have no clinical significance when plain films are normal [69]. Pelvic ultrasound is important to exclude an intrauterine pregnancy or retained trophoblastic tissue from incomplete uterine evacuation of a molar pregnancy [41,43]. In many algorithms, a CT of the abdomen and brain are included as baseline studies, but it is also reasonable not to obtain all of these studies for patients with a normal history and physical examination, normal chest radiograph and chest CT, and low pretreatment hCG titer ($<40,000$ mIU/mL) [65]. Patients with histologically proven PSTT should be classified separately from those with choriocarcinoma or postmolar GTN [4].

Although rates vary significantly by race and ethnicity, geographic region, and maternal age, molar pregnancies are relatively common, and affect 1 in 850 pregnancies in the United States and North America [28,70,71]. Therefore, the practicing gynecologist is likely to encounter and should be able to diagnose and manage uncomplicated GTD and provide postmolar surveillance. However, because the prognosis of patients with GTN is dependent upon thorough assessment of risk, it is strongly advocated that patients be referred to a regional referral center or gynecologic oncologist experienced in the management of this condition in complicated GTD cases or if the patient meets the criteria for GTN [54,72]. Although choriocarcinoma incidence rates have declined in the United States by almost 50% over the past 25 years, in the most recent 5-year period analyzed (1993–1997), rates had actually increased. This trend may be a reflection of fewer referrals to centers that specialize in the management of this relatively rare disease [28].

Prophylactic chemotherapy has been evaluated in selected patients who have complete mole, to reduce the risk of GTN and to shorten the surveillance interval. In high-risk patients, a single dose of methotrexate followed by folic acid reduced the incidence of post-molar GTN from 47.4% to 14.3%, but no benefit was achieved in low-risk patients [73]. Comparable results have also been reported using actinomycin D [74]. Although no patients in either of these prospective trials died of complications, deaths attributable to prophylactic chemotherapy have been reported [75]. Therefore, we do not advocate use of prophylactic chemotherapy in patients with GTD because (1) chemotherapy does not eliminate the need for surveillance, (2) use of chemotherapy in patients who subsequently develop GTN increases the risk of drug resistance, (3) there will be patients who receive cytotoxic chemotherapy in whom the disease would have responded spontaneously, and (4) chemotherapy is not without risk.

## Low-risk gestational trophoblastic neoplasia

Patients with low-risk GTN are patients who have non-metastatic or metastatic GTN to the lung or vagina only, and a FIGO risk score of less than 7 (Table 2). Treatment for low-risk GTN is single-agent chemotherapy using one of the following regimens.

Methotrexate 1 mg/kg intramuscular (IM) on days 1, 3, 5, and 7, with folinic acid 0.1 mg/kg IM on days 2, 4, 6, and 8; repeat every 7 days if possible.

Methotrexate 0.4 mg/kg (20–25 mg) intravenous (IV) or IM daily for 5 days; repeat every 7 days if possible. If no response, increase dose to 0.6 mg/kg or switch to actinomycin D.

Methotrexate 40 mg/M2 IM weekly.

Actinomycin D 12 µg/kg IV daily for 5 days; repeat every 7 days. If no response, add 2 µg/kg to the initial dose or switch to methotrexate.

Pulse actinomycin D: 1.25 mg/M2; repeat every 2 weeks.

Oral methotrexate alternating with folinic acid has been used with a 90% response rate [76], but intramuscular or intravenous dosing of methotrexate is preferred by most experts to ensure compliance and to avoid variable absorption. Phase II studies of weekly methotrexate by the Gynecology Oncology Group (GOG) found that dose levels of 30, 40, and 50 mg/M$^2$ are comparable in efficacy and toxicity; a median efficacy of 77.6% and 7 cycles are needed to sustain remission [77]. Methotrexate is not recommended for patients with significant liver dysfunction. Initially used as a 5-day regimen, "pulsed" actinomycin D given every other week has a 92% response rate, is inexpensive, and has less nausea and alopecia than the daily 5-day course of infusion [78]. On the other hand, it has also been reported that "pulsed" regimens have a higher failure rate than 5-day actinomycin D, and that 60% of patients who fail the "pulse" therapy respond to a 5-day schedule of the same drug. This suggests that trophoblastic cells need longer exposure to the medication and that the 5-day course permits more cells to be in cycle [79]. Because actinomycin D is a potent vesicant, administration should be through a fresh, free-flowing intravenous peripheral line or central venous catheter. A prospective randomized GOG trial (#174) is ongoing to determine the difference in cost, response, and toxicity of weekly methotrexate and pulsed actinomycin D in low-risk GTD. Oral etoposide, a topoisomerase II inhibitor, is highly active against choriocarcinoma, and has a relapse rate of only 1 in 60 patients [80]. However, etoposide always causes alopecia. Of even greater concern, etoposide in combination with alkylating agents increases the risk of treatment-related myelodysplasia/leukemia [81]. For this reason, this agent has lost favor as primary treatment for low-risk disease. In one study, the 40-month cumulative incidence of myelodysplasia/leukemia was 8%, which was significantly higher than the expected number in this patient group, 0.001%. Nevertheless, because actinomycin D in methotrexate-refractory GTN has limited activity [82], singe-agent etoposide may play a role in this setting [83–85], especially in women under 39 years of age who want to remain fertile [85]. The pyrimidine analong 5-fluorouracil (5-FU) is commonly used in Asia for metastatic and non-metastatic GTN, and response rates as high as 94% have been reported in low-risk disease. In high-risk disease, the response rate of 5-FU combined with nitrocaphanum was 73.3% [86], and in patients with etoposide–refractory disease, 80% combined with actinomycin D. However, because of its pharmacokinetic and toxicity profile (5-FU is most effective given as a continuous infusion over 10 days, and is associated with gastrointestinal and bone marrow toxicity), in the United States this agent is usually reserved for refractory cases only [87,88].

For low-risk GTN, usually one additional dose of therapy is given after the hCG titer normalizes. The biological rational of this is the following: 1 cm$^3$ of tumor contains $10^9$ cancer cells. hCG disappears from serum at $10^7$ cells. Therefore, this additional chemotherapy is given to eradicate clinically undetectable cells. In one series, the rate of recurrence following molar pregnancy was 2.5% (5 of 204 patients with non-metastatic GTN), and all were within 36 months of initial treatment: 50% within 3 months, and 85% within 18 months. Recurrence was strongly linked to inadequate staging, non-compliance with chemotherapy once the hCG titer normalized, and delays between scheduled cycles of therapy. However, half of the patients in this series had a second recurrence, and of these, 45% had a third recurrence [89]. This emphasizes the need for continued surveillance in patients who are in clinical remission (usually defined as three normal weekly hCG titers).

The overall cure rate for patients with low-risk GTN is close to 100%. Hysterectomy is an alternative to shorten the duration of chemotherapy in patients who have completed childbearing, but does not replace the need for postmolar surveillance. In patients with isolated refractory disease in the uterus, hysterectomy may be indicated; pulmonary metastases have similarly been salvaged by partial lobectomy or segmental resection [90–92].

## High risk gestational trophoblastic neoplasia

Patients who have GTN metastatic to the brain, liver, or sites other than lung and vagina, and who have a FIGO risk score greater than 7—which is based upon the number and location of lesions and prior chemotherapy (Fig. 2)— have high-risk GTN. Treatment includes using multiagent chemotherapy, surgery, or radiation therapy [89,93–95]. High-risk GTN survival rates from regional trophoblastic disease centers approach 84%, even in women with brain metastases [96–102]. Any patient with pulmonary metastases on a chest radiograph and chest CT scan, should have a complete evaluation as previously outlined for low-risk GTN. In addition, they should have an MRI of the brain and CT scan of the abdomen and pelvis. Hematuria can be indicative of renal metastasis, which can be evaluated further by intravenous pyelography [103,104]. Because hCG does not readily diffuse across the blood-brain barrier, patients with brain metastases may have elevated cerebral spinal fluid hCG relative to serum hCG levels. A cerebrospinal fluid (CSF)/serum beta-hCG ratio >1:60 suggests but is not diagnostic for intracranial metastases; patients with ratios <1:60 and brain metastases have been reported. However, this immunomarker can serve as a valuable monitoring tool when patients have no radiographic evidence of neurological involvement [101,105–107].

Multiple-agent chemotherapy is the treatment of choice for patients with high-risk GTN. For many years, the standard treatment of metastatic GTN was triple drug therapy using methotrexate, actinomycin D, and chlorambucil or cyclophosphamide (the MAC regimen), which had a 60% response rate but significant toxicity. A randomized trial by the GOG determined that MAC was as effective as the more commonly used Bagshawe regimen, but was less toxic. The introduction of etoposide in 1982 dramatically changed the current approach to high-risk GTN. The regimen currently recommended as the treatment of choice for high-risk metastatic GTN is EMA-CO chemotherapy (Box 1).

In patients with central nervous system metastases, the dose of methotrexate should be increased to 1.0 $g/m^2$ as a 24-hour infusion, and the folinic acid increased to 15 mg orally or intravenously every 8 hours × 9 doses, beginning after completion of methotrexate infusion. Patients with central nervous system metastases or high-risk FIGO prognostic index scores, may also receive methotrexate, 12.5 mg, by intrathecal injection. When given in high does, methotrexate

---

**Box 1. EMA-CO chemotherapy for high-risk GTN**

*Course 1 (EMA)*

Day 1
Etoposide 100 $mg/m^2$, IV infusion in 200 mL normal saline
Actinomycin D 0.5 mg, IV push
Methotrexate 100 $mg/m^2$ push followed by 200 $mg/m^2$, IV over 12 hours
Day 2
Etoposide 100 $mg/m^2$ IV infusion in 200 mL normal saline over 30 minutes
Actinomycin D 0.5 mg IV push
Folinic acid, 15 mg IM or orally every 12 hours for 4 courses 24 hours after start of methotrexate

*Course 2 (CO)*

Day 8
Vincristine sulfate (Oncovin), 1.0 $mg/m^2$, IV push
Cyclophosphamide (Cytoxan), 600 $mg/m^2$, IV infusion

can be nephrotoxic, as 90% is excreted unchanged in the urine. Therefore, use of sodium bicarbonate to maintain urinary pH > 7 can protect against renal tubule precipitation. High rates of success have been reported with this regimen [108–110]; however, recent reports of leukemia in survivors mandate critical appraisal on an individual basis of risks versus benefits [81,111–114].

The ideal management of intracranial metastasis is controversial. The patient should be evaluated for medical and radiographic evidence of neurological impairment or bleeding and may require intracranial exploration to survive. Steroids may be required to reduce cerebral edema. Most series recommend systemic and intrathecal methotrexate in combination with whole brain irradiation therapy to reduce the risk of intracranial bleeding, although comparable survival rates have also been reported with high-dose chemotherapy without brain radiation. Subacute demyelinating syndrome following intracranial methotrexate and whole-brain irradiation therapy has been reported following this regimen, especially in young children, and when 3000 centigray (cGy) is given in 300 cGy fractions. There are also no universal guidelines for liver metastases. Radiation therapy (2000 cGy) has been advocated to reduce the risk of bleeding in addition to multiagent chemotherapy, but as for other sites of metastasis, surgery may be necessary to control hemorrhage or remove chemo-resistant disease. Typically, two or three cycles of chemotherapy are given after achieving complete remission. Salvage of chemo-resistant disease has been reported with bleomycin, cisplatin, and etoposide [115], high-dose chemotherapy and stem cell support [114,116], ifosfamide alone or in combination with other agents [115,117–120], and more recently, with paclitaxel [121–124]. These newer studies indicate a need to compare paclitaxel/platin-containing regimens with etoposide-based combinations in this setting [122–126]. Liver metastases not responding to EMA-CO or EMA-EP chemotherapy may respond to surgical resection arterial embolization, or antevial chemotherapy.

## Gestational trophoblastic neoplasia and pregnancy

*Risk factors for developing molar pregnancy and implications for future pregnancies*

For future pregnancies, there is a 10-fold increased risk (1%–2%) of a second hydatidiform mole, and with early ultrasound a subsequent prognosis is advocated. Maternal age has consistently been identified as an important risk factor. Age-specific incidence reports usually reveal a 'J curve' and teenagers <18 years old and women >40 have higher rates, probably secondary to defects in ovoid function. A higher rate of hydatidiform mole (HM) after artificial insemination by donor has also been reported [127], as well as repetitive molar pregnancies with different male partners. Family clusters have been reported, indicating rare familial patterns. Patients should be reassured that most patients with low-risk GTD have favorable reproductive outcomes. Data with respect to future fertility following chemotherapy for GTN is cautiously optimistic, but long-term data regarding potential effects upon the unborn child, particularly with etoposide, are unknown. However, the patient can be assured that for herself, leukemia is rare following pulsed therapy and less than 7 courses of EMA-CO.

*Hydatidiform mole coexisting with a twin live fetus*

Twin pregnancies with a hydatidiform mole and an apparently normal fetus affect 0.01% to 0.001% of all pregnancies [128]. The differential diagnosis includes a triploid singleton gestation, a twin pregnancy with CM, and a twin pregnancy with a PM. Usually, twin pregnancies with CM and normal fetus have a molar pregnancy attached or separated from a normal placenta. Twins with PM typically show a triploid molar placenta and a normal placenta, have fewer hydropic villa and lower hCG levels. Presenting symptoms of CM–fetal twin gestations include bleeding, escalated uterine growth, and early onset pre-eclampsia. Compared with PM–twin gestations, CM–twin gestations tend to be diagnosed at a later EGA and have higher hCG levels. The karyotype of the fetus may be normal or abnormal, and therefore expertise in cytogenetics is invaluable to guide counseling with respect to continuing the pregnancy. Very rarely, twins with both PM and CM have been reported [129], and rarer still, transformation of a monozygotic twin into PM [130]. In many cases, the diagnosis of a HM–twin is suggested by symptoms and is made on ultrasound before delivery, but in about a third, the only definite ultrasonic abnormality is a uterine mass [128,131]. In one case, the diagnosis was suspected because an empty gestational sack was seen at 7 weeks but was not seen on later ultrasounds [131]. Several authors have reported CM–twin gestations after the use of clomiphene or hMG-hCG therapy [128,132–134]. However, gestational trophoblastic disease is a complication of in vitro fertilization [135,136] and has been reported in women undergoing artificial insemination [127,137]. This suggests that ovulation induction is an independent risk factor for both twins and GTN.

There are no accepted guidelines for the management of twin–molar pregnancies. Case reports from the 1970s through the 1990s emphasized a high rate of persistent GTN and poor fetal outcome. Since then, a significant portion of these pregnancies are terminated for medical indications [138–140]. Stellar and colleagues [138] found that 5 of 8 CM–twin gestations developed persistent GTD which required chemotherapy; of these, 3 developed metastases that required combination chemotherapy to achieve remission. They concluded that CM–twins tended to be diagnosed at a later gestation, had higher preevacuation β-hCG levels, and were at high risk for developing persistent GTN. Another two cases of twin pregnancies with CM with intent to preserve the pregnancies ended with normal infants delivered at 41 and 26 weeks EGA. Including these two cases, the authors identified 15 CM–twin pregnancies in the literature between 1977 and 1999 where pregnancy was allowed to continue. Of these, 8 (55.3%) developed GTN and 4 (27.7%), metastatic disease [128]. In another series, two cases were complicated by severe preeclampsia that resulted in pregnancy termination: 1 at 16 weeks EGA for this condition and thyrotoxicosis, and 1 by cesarean delivery at 26 weeks for an infant who did not survive [131].

Perhaps the best recommendations can be garnered from data reported by centers that have consistently maintained a centralized database on GTN [141]. In a national collaborative study conducted in Japan, 72 cases of HM–twins were identified, 18 cytogenetically confirmed CM. The risk overall of persistent GTN was 30.6%, and increased to 50% in the 18 patients who had CM–twins. The incidence of maternal complications such as preeclampsia and uterine bleeding was higher in the nine patients who continued their pregnancies. However, there was no difference in the incidence of GTN with advancing duration of pregnancy, and the authors concluded that continued pregnancy may be feasible [142]. The largest series to date of HM and healthy co-twin, 126 cases, was reported from the Charing Cross Hospital Trophoblastic Disease Unit. Of these, 77 had CM, and 49 had partial moles. Management of the 77 CM cases was as follows: 19 underwent elective termination before week 14, 5 between week 15 and 22, and 53 elected to continue the pregnancy. Of these, 2 terminated the pregnancy for preeclampsia before week 24; 23 underwent spontaneous abortion or intrauterine death before week 24; and 28 delivered at 24 weeks or later. Of cases where the pregnancy continued, there was 1 neonatal death, 7 intrauterine deaths, and 20 live births. Chemotherapy to eliminate GTN was required in 3 of 19 patients (16%) who terminated their pregnancy in the first trimester, and 12 of 58 (21%) who continued their pregnancies. While these data indicate a high risk of spontaneous abortion, about 40% resulted in live births, without significantly increasing the risk of post delivery GTN. Of the 15 patients with post partum GTN, single agent chemotherapy was curative in 3/3 women who terminated pregnancy and in 7/12 who allowed their pregnancies to continue, 4 of whom eventually required multiagent chemotherapy. All were cured of their disease (median follow up 12 years). In this series, there were two fetal deaths from placental mesenchymal dysplasia, one at 16-18 weeks EGA, and the other 24–35 weeks EGA. One infant developed necrotizing enterocolitis at 28 weeks but survived. Of the pregnancies that continued past 24 weeks, only one woman developed severe preeclampsia, and required delivery at 29 weeks. One patient experienced a pulmonary embolus after vaginal delivery that was not associated with the development of post partum GTN. These data demonstrate that a high rate of fetal mortality (60%) can be expected, excluding elective terminations. However, these data show that up to 40% of women can expect to deliver live babies beyond 32 weeks EGA without significantly increasing their risks of post partum GTN [143]. This series and others [128,131] confirm the risk of severe preeclampsia and twin–mole gestation, but in this large series the risk was 6%. [143]. By way of comparison, the rate of preeclampsia in singleton pregnancies in one large series was 3.19% (eclampsia 0.04%) compared with 9.25% (eclampsia 0.16%) in twin pregnancies [144]. Therefore, although rates of preeclampsia are higher in HM compared with singleton gestations, they are not necessarily elevated with HM–twins relative to other twin gestations.

Based upon these data, we recommend that patients who choose to continue the pregnancy be cared for by a team with collective expertise in high-risk pregnancy and gestational trophoblastic disease management. Although they may be inaccurate in making the diagnosis in a third of cases, serial ultrasounds are warranted for fetal surveillance. Determination of fetal karyotype by cytogenetics is invaluable. Patients must be informed of the added risks of preeclampsia, tyrotoxicosis, intrauterine growth retardation, premature delivery, and GTD spread. A chest radiograph to assess for pulmonary metastasis is appropriate, and if positive, a comprehensive workup including MRI of the chest, abdomen, and pelvis. The diagnosis of choriocarcinoma complicating a viable pregnancy is exceedlingly rare; typically, these patients present with neurological manifestations or hemorrhage. Time is critical; in these patients, staging prompt, appropriate therapy is imperative without regard to the fetus [145–147].

## Pregnancy following chemotherapy for gestational trophoblastic neoplasia

In most situations, patients with a history of molar pregnancy can expect to maintain normal reproductive function, with risks of stillbirth and reproductive success comparable to the general population [148]. However, patients who have had a molar pregnancy have an increased risk of 1% to 2% for a second mole, and should undergo ultrasound as soon as pregnancy is suspected [149–151]. Occasionally women become pregnant before completing 6 months of hCG surveillance. Although the vast majority of these can expect to have a normal outcome, like any other patient under post-molar surveillance, there is a low but real risk for GTN; at least one case of choriocarcinoma coincident with the pregnancy under these circumstances has been reported [152]. Fertility is usually spared following single-agent chemotherapy; however, multi-agent chemotherapy with alkylating agents and cisplatin increases the risk for oligomenorrhea, and at least theoretically this can have an impact on further fertility. Despite this, at least one case of a successful pregnancy after EMA-CO chemotherapy has been reported [150]. Long-term data are needed to determine if there is any late effect of chemotherapy on the offspring of these women.

## Summary

Throughout the world, the rates of GTN and choriocarcinoma are decreasing and survival has dramatically improved [28,70]. We now have improved guidelines to delineate more clearly those patients who should undergo treatment and who should be observed, and an improved FIGO staging system that combines FIGO staging with the modified Charing Cross/WHO risk factor scoring system. With low-risk GTN, survival approaches 100%. Appropriate surveillance is essential, as is timely and complete treatment with chemotherapy as indicated by risk-factor score. For patients with high-risk disease, and even those with choriocarcinoma, the prognosis is favorable with timely, appropriate staging and chemotherapy. Patients with a previous molar pregnancy should have an ultrasound to rule out another mole in subequent pregnancies, but except in rare circumstances such as familial GTN [135,136,153], they can expect to sustain normal pregnancies. The most important factors to assure successful therapy, as illustrated by the central referral practiced in the United Kingdom, are knowledge and experience with GTN and GTD, a reliable hCG assay, experience with chemotherapy, and patient compliance.

## References

[1] ACOG Committee on Practice Bulletins. Practice Bulletin #53. Diagnosis and treatment of gestational trophoblastic disease. Obstet Gynecol 2004;104:1422–3.

[2] Benedet JL, Bender H, Jones 3rd H, et al. FIGO staging classifications and clinical practice guidelines in the management of gynecologic cancers. Int J Gynaecol Obstet 2000;70(2): 209–62.

[3] Kohorn EI. Negotiating a staging and risk factor scoring system for gestational trophoblastic neoplasia. A progress report. J Reprod Med 2002;47(6):445–50.

[4] Kohorn EI. The new FIGO 2000 staging and risk factor scoring system for gestational trophoblastic disease: description and critical assessment. Int J Gynecol Cancer 2001;11(1): 73–7.

[5] Soto-Wright V, Bernstein M, Goldstein DP, et al. The changing clinical presentation of complete molar pregnancy. Obstet Gynecol 1995;86(5):775–9.

[6] Mosher R, Goldstein DP, Berkowitz R, et al. Complete hydatidiform mole. Comparison of clinicopathologic features, current and past. J Reprod Med 1998;43(1):21–7.

[7] Kajii T, Ohama K. Androgenetic origin of hydatidiform mole. Nature 1977;268(5621):633–4.

[8] Kajii T. The road to diploid androgenesis (the Japan Society of Human Genetics award lecture). Jinrui Idengaku Zasshi 1986;31(2):61–71.

[9] Kajii T, Kurashige H, Ohama K, et al. XY and XX complete moles: clinical and morphologic correlations. Am J Obstet Gynecol 1984;150(1):57–64.

[10] Wake N, Takagi N, Sasaki M. Androgenesis as a cause of hydatidiform mole. J Natl Cancer Inst 1978;60(1):51–7.

[11] Ohama K, Kajii T, Okamoto E, et al. Dispermic origin of XY hydatidiform moles. Nature 1981;292(5823):551–2.

[12] Bewtra C, Frankforter S, Marcus JN. Clinicopathologic differences between diploid and tetraploid complete hydatidiform moles. Int J Gynecol Pathol 1997;16(3):239–44.

[13] Shigematsu T, Kamura T, Saito T, et al. Identification of persistent trophoblastic diseases based on a human chorionic gonadotropin regression curve by means of a stepwise piecewise linear regression analysis after the evacuation of uneventful moles. Gynecol Oncol 1998;71(3): 376–80.

[14] Genest DR. Partial hydatidiform mole: clinicopathological features, differential diagnosis, ploidy and molecular studies, and gold standards for diagnosis. Int J Gynecol Pathol 2001; 20(4):315–22.

[15] Lage JM, Wolf NG. Gestational trophoblastic disease. New approaches to diagnosis. Clin Lab Med 1995;15(3):631–64.

[16] Szulman AE, Philippe E, Boue JG, et al. Human triploidy: association with partial hydatidiform moles and nonmolar conceptuses. Hum Pathol 1981;12(11):1016–21.

[17] Szulman AE, Surti U. The syndromes of hydatidiform mole. II. Morphologic evolution of the complete and partial mole. Am J Obstet Gynecol 1978;132(1):20–7.

[18] Jeffers MD, Michie BA, Oakes SJ, et al. Comparison of ploidy analysis by flow cytometry and

image analysis in hydatidiform mole and non-molar abortion. Histopathology 1995;27(5): 415–21.

[19] Jeffers MD, O'Dwyer P, Curran B, et al. Partial hydatidiform mole: a common but underdiagnosed condition. A 3-year retrospective clinicopathological and DNA flow cytometric analysis. Int J Gynecol Pathol 1993;12(4):315–23.

[20] Bocklage TJ, Smith HO, Bartow SA. Distinctive flow histogram pattern in molar pregnancies with elevated maternal serum human chorionic gonadotropin levels. Cancer 1994;73(11): 2782–90.

[21] Lage JM, Bagg A. Hydatidiform moles: DNA flow cytometry, image analysis and selected topics in molecular biology. Histopathology 1996;28(4):379–82.

[22] Seckl MJ, Fisher RA, Salerno G, et al. Choriocarcinoma and partial hydatidiform moles. Lancet 2000;356(9223):36–9.

[23] Cheung AN, Khoo US, Lai CY, et al. Metastatic trophoblastic disease after an initial diagnosis of partial hydatidiform mole: genotyping and chromosome in situ hybridization analysis. Cancer 2004;100(7):1411–7.

[24] Menczer J, Girtler O, Zajdel L, et al. Metastatic trophoblastic disease following partial hydatidiform mole: case report and literature review. Gynecol Oncol 1999;74(2):304–7.

[25] Smith HO, Qualls CR, Hilgers RD, et al. Gestational trophoblastic neoplasia in American Indians. J Reprod Med 2004;49(7):535–44.

[26] Bentley RC. Pathology of gestational trophoblastic disease. Clin Obstet Gynecol 2003;46(3): 513–22.

[27] Suzuki T, Goto S, Nawa A, et al. Identification of the pregnancy responsible for gestational trophoblastic disease by DNA analysis. Obstet Gynecol 1993;82(4 Pt 1):629–34.

[28] Smith HO, Qualls CR, Prairie BA, et al. Trends in gestational choriocarcinoma: a 27-year perspective. Obstet Gynecol 2003;102(5 Pt 1):978–87.

[29] Bracken MB, Brinton LA, Hayashi K. Epidemiology of hydatidiform mole and choriocarcinoma. Epidemiol Rev 1984;6:52–75.

[30] Brinton LA, Bracken MB, Connelly RR. Choriocarcinoma incidence in the United States. Am J Epidemiol 1986;123(6):1094–100.

[31] Shanmugaratnam K, Muir CS, Tow SH, et al. Rates per 100,000 births and incidence of choriocarcinoma and malignant mole in Singapore Chinese and Malays. Comparison with Connecticut, Norway and Sweden. Int J Cancer 1971;8(1):165–75.

[32] Yingna S, Yang X, Xiuyu Y, et al. Clinical characteristics and treatment of gestational trophoblastic tumor with vaginal metastasis. Gynecol Oncol 2002;84(3):416–9.

[33] Horn LC, Bilek K. Clinicopathologic analysis of gestational trophoblastic disease–report of 158 cases. Gen Diagn Pathol 1997;143(2–3):173–8.

[34] Lurain JR, Casanova LA, Miller DS, et al. Prognostic factors in gestational trophoblastic tumors: a proposed new scoring system based on multivariate analysis. Am J Obstet Gynecol 1991;164(2):611–6.

[35] Jacques SM, Qureshi F, Doss BJ, et al. Intraplacental choriocarcinoma associated with viable pregnancy: pathologic features and implications for the mother and infant. Pediatr Dev Pathol 1998;1(5):380–7.

[36] Suh YK. Placental pathology casebook. Choriocarcinoma in situ of placenta associated with transplacental hemorrhage. J Perinatol 1999;19(2):153–4.

[37] Feltmate CM, Genest DR, Goldstein DP, et al. Advances in the understanding of placental site trophoblastic tumor. J Reprod Med 2002;47(5):337–41.

[38] Kim SJ. Placental site trophoblastic tumour. Best Pract Res Clin Obstet Gynaecol 2003; 17(6):969–84.

[39] Machtinger R, Gotlieb WH, Korach J, et al. Placental site trophoblastic tumor: outcome of five cases including fertility preserving management. Gynecol Oncol 2005;96(1):56–61.

[40] Papadopoulos AJ, Foskett M, Seckl MJ, et al. Twenty-five years' clinical experience with placental site trophoblastic tumors. J Reprod Med 2002;47(6):460–4.

[41] Jauniaux E. Ultrasound diagnosis and follow-up of gestational trophoblastic disease. Ultrasound Obstet Gynecol 1998;11(5):367–77.

[42] Bidzinski M, Lemieszczuk B, Drabik M. The assessment of value of transvaginal ultrasound for monitoring of gestational trophoblastic disease treatment. Eur J Gynaecol Oncol 1997;18(6): 541–3.

[43] Goldstein DP, Garner EI, Feltmate CM, et al. The role of repeat uterine evacuation in the management of persistent gestational trophoblastic disease. Gynecol Oncol 2004;95(3):421–2.

[44] Amir SM, Osathanondh R, Berkowitz RS, et al. Human chorionic gonadotropin and thyroid function in patients with hydatidiform mole. Am J Obstet Gynecol 1984;150(6):723–8.

[45] Hershman JM. Physiological and pathological aspects of the effect of human chorionic gonadotropin on the thyroid. Best Pract Res Clin Endocrinol Metab 2004;18(2):249–65.

[46] Hershman JM. Human chorionic gonadotropin and the thyroid: hyperemesis gravidarum and trophoblastic tumors. Thyroid 1999;9(7):653–7.

[47] Elmer DB, Granai CO, Ball HG, et al. Persistence of gestational trophoblastic disease for longer than 1 year following evacuation of hydatidiform mole. Obstet Gynecol 1993;81(5 Pt 2): 888–90.

[48] Wolfberg AJ, Feltmate C, Goldstein DP, et al. Low risk of relapse after achieving undetectable HCG levels in women with complete molar pregnancy. Obstet Gynecol 2004;104(3):551–4.

[49] Parazzini F, Cipriani S, Mangili G, et al. Oral contraceptives and risk of gestational tropho-blastic disease. Contraception 2002;65(6):425–7.

[50] Stone M, Bagshawe KD. An analysis of the influences of maternal age, gestational age, contraceptive method, and the mode of primary treatment of patients with hydatidiform moles on the incidence of subsequent chemotherapy. Br J Obstet Gynaecol 1979;86(10):782–92.

[51] Palmer JR, Driscoll SG, Rosenberg L, et al. Oral contraceptive use and risk of gestational trophoblastic tumors. J Natl Cancer Inst 1999;91(7):635–40.

[52] Curry SL, Schlaerth JB, Kohorn EI, et al. Hormonal contraception and trophoblastic sequelae after hydatidiform mole. Am J Obstet Gynecol 1989;160(4):805–9 [discussion 809–11].

[53] Morrow P, Nakamura R, Schlaerth J, et al. The influence of oral contraceptives on the post-molar human chorionic gonadotropin regression curve. Am J Obstet Gynecol 1985;151(7): 906–14.

[54] Guidelines for referral to a gynecologic oncologist: rationale and benefits. The Society of Gynecologic Oncologists. Gynecol Oncol 2000;78(3 Pt 2):S1–13.

[55] Cole LA, Khanlian SA. Inappropriate management of women with persistent low hCG results. J Reprod Med 2004;49(6):423–32.

[56] Khanlian SA, Smith HO, Cole LA. Persistent low levels of human chorionic gonadotropin: a premalignant gestational trophoblastic disease. Am J Obstet Gynecol 2003;188(5):1254–9.

[57] Newlands E. Presentation and management of persistent gestational trophoblastic disease (GTD) and gestational trophoblastic tumors (GTT) in the United Kingdom. In: Handcock BW NE, Berkowitz RS, Cole LA, editors. Gestational Trophoblastic Disease. 2nd Edition. Sheffield, United Kingdom: Sheffield Universtiy Press; 2003. p. 229–47.

[58] Handcock BW, Tidy J. Clinical management of persistent low level hCG elevation. Trophoblastic Disease Update 2002;4:5–6.

[59] Kohorn EI. What we know about low-level hCG: definition, classification and management. J Reprod Med 2004;49(6):433–7.

[60] Kohorn EI. Persistent low-level "real" human chorionic gonadotropin: a clinical challenge and a therapeutic dilemma. Gynecol Oncol 2002;85(2):315–20.

[61] Newlands E. Presentation and management of persistent gestational trophoblastic disease (GTD) and gestational trophoblastic tumours (GTT) in the United Kingdom. In: Hancock BW, Newlands ES, Berkowitz RS, Cole LA, editors. Gestational trophoblastic disease. 2nd edition. Sheffield, United Kingdom: International Society for the Study of Trophoblastic Diseases; 2003. p. 229–47.

[62] Cole LA. Phantom hCG and phantom choriocarcinoma. Gynecol Oncol 1998;71(2):325–9.

[63] ACOG. Committee opinion: number 278, November 2002. Avoiding inappropriate clinical decisions based on false-positive human chorionic gonadotropin test results. Obstet Gynecol 2002;100(5 Pt 1):1057–9.

[64] Soper JT. Staging and evaluation of gestational trophoblastic disease. Clin Obstet Gynecol 2003;46(3):570–8.

[65] Hunter V, Raymond E, Christensen C, et al. Efficacy of the metastatic survey in the staging of gestational trophoblastic disease. Cancer 1990;65(7):1647–50.

[66] Mutch DG, Soper JT, Baker ME, et al. Role of computed axial tomography of the chest in staging patients with nonmetastatic gestational trophoblastic disease. Obstet Gynecol 1986; 68(3):348–52.

[67] Moodley M, Moodley J. Evaluation of chest X-ray findings to determine metastatic gestational trophoblastic disease according to the proposed new staging system: a case series. J Obstet Gynaecol 2004;24(3):287–8.

[68] Gamer EI, Garrett A, Goldstein DP, et al. Significance of chest computed tomography findings in the evaluation and treatment of persistent gestational trophoblastic neoplasia. J Reprod Med 2004;49(6):411–4.

[69] Ngan HY, Chan FL, Au VW, et al. Clinical outcome of micrometastasis in the lung in stage IA persistent gestational trophoblastic disease. Gynecol Oncol 1998;70(2):192–4.

[70] Smith HO. Gestational trophoblastic disease epidemiology and trends. Clin Obstet Gynecol 2003;46(3):541–56.

[71] Smith HO, Hilgers RD, Bedrick EJ, et al. Ethnic differences at risk for gestational trophoblastic disease in New Mexico: a 25-year population-based study. Am J Obstet Gynecol 2003;188(2):357–66.

[72] Soper JT, Evans AC, Conaway MR, et al. Evaluation of prognostic factors and staging in gestational trophoblastic tumor. Obstet Gynecol 1994;84(6):969–73.

[73] Kim DS, Moon H, Kim KT, et al. Effects of prophylactic chemotherapy for persistent trophoblastic disease in patients with complete hydatidiform mole. Obstet Gynecol 1986; 67(5):690–4.

[74] Limpongsanurak S. Prophylactic actinomycin D for high-risk complete hydatidiform mole. J Reprod Med 2001;46(2):110–6.

[75] Curry SL, Hammond CB, Tyrey L, et al. Hydatidiform mole: diagnosis, management, and long-term followup of 347 patients. Obstet Gynecol 1975;45(1):1–8.

[76] Berkowitz RS, Goldstein DP, Bernstein MR. Methotrexate with citrovorum factor rescue as primary therapy for gestational trophoblastic disease. Cancer 1982;50(10):2024–7.

[77] Homesley HD, Blessing JA, Schlaerth J, et al. Rapid escalation of weekly intramuscular methotrexate for nonmetastatic gestational trophoblastic disease. Gynecol Oncol 1990;39(3): 305–8.

[78] Petrilli ES, Twiggs LB, Blessing JA, et al. Single-dose actinomycin-D treatment for nonmetastatic gestational trophoblastic disease. A prospective phase II trial of the Gynecologic Oncology Group. Cancer 1987;60(9):2173–6.

[79] Kohorn EI. Is lack of response to single-agent chemotherapy in gestational trophoblastic disease associated with dose scheduling or chemotherapy resistance? Gynecol Oncol 2002;85(1):36–9.

[80] Wong LC, Choo YC, Ma HK. Use of oral VP16-213 as primary chemotherapeutic agent in treatment of gestational trophoblastic disease. Am J Obstet Gynecol 1984;150(8):924–7.

[81] Akyol D, Mungan T, Baltaci V, et al. Clinical assessment of EMA/CO induced DNA damage in peripheral blood lymphocytes of high-risk gestational trophoblastic tumor patients. Eur J Gynaecol Oncol 1999;20(2):150–5.

[82] Chen LM, Lengyel ER, Bethan Powell C. Single-agent pulse dactinomycin has only modest activity for methotrexate-resistant gestational trophoblastic neoplasia. Gynecol Oncol 2004;94(1):204–7.

[83] Matsui H, Iitsuka Y, Seki K, et al. Comparison of chemotherapies with methotrexate, VP-16 and actinomycin-D in low-risk gestational trophoblastic disease. Remission rates and drug toxicities. Gynecol Obstet Invest 1998;46(1):5–8.

[84] Mangili G, Garavaglia E, Frigerio L, et al. Management of low-risk gestational trophoblastic tumors with etoposide (VP16) in patients resistant to methotrexate. Gynecol Oncol 1996;61(2):218–20.

[85] Matsui H, Seki K, Sekiya S, et al. Reproductive status in GTD treated with etoposide. J Reprod Med 1997;42(2):104–10.

[86] Wang Y, Jiu L, Guan Y, et al. Chemotherapy using 5-fluorouracil and nitrocaphanum in malignant trophoblastic tumor. Gynecol Oncol 1998;71(3):416–9.

[87] Matsui H, Suzuka K, Iitsuka Y, et al. Salvage combination chemotherapy with 5-fluorouracil and actinomycin D for patients with refractory, high-risk gestational trophoblastic tumors. Cancer 2002;95(5):1051–4.

[88] Sung HC, Wu PC, Yang HY. Reevaluation of 5-fluorouracil as a single therapeutic agent for gestational trophoblastic neoplasms. Am J Obstet Gynecol 1984;150(1):69–75.

[89] Mutch DG, Soper JT, Babcock CJ, et al. Recurrent gestational trophoblastic disease. Experience of the Southeastern Regional Trophoblastic Disease Center. Cancer 1990;66(5):978–82.

[90] Carlson N, Winter 3rd WE, Krivak TC, et al. Successful management of metastatic placental site trophoblastic tumor with multiple pulmonary resections. Gynecol Oncol 2002;87(1): 146–9.

[91] Lehman E, Gershenson DM, Burke TW, et al. Salvage surgery for chemorefractory gestational trophoblastic disease. J Clin Oncol 1994;12(12):2737–42.

[92] Suzuka K, Matsui H, Iitsuka Y, et al. Adjuvant hysterectomy in low-risk gestational trophoblastic disease. Obstet Gynecol 2001;97(3):431–4.

[93] Bilgin T, Ozan H, Ozuysal S, et al. Successful salvage therapy of resistant gestational trophoblastic disease with etoposide, methotrexate, actinomycin-D, etoposide, cisplatin (EMA/EP). Arch Gynecol Obstet 2004;269(2):159–60.

[94] Kim SJ, Bae SN, Kim JH, et al. Effects of multiagent chemotherapy and independent risk factors in the treatment of high-risk GTT–25 years experiences of KRI-TRD. Int J Gynaecol Obstet 1998;60(Suppl 1):S85–96.

[95] Crawford RA, Newlands E, Rustin GJ, et al. Gestational trophoblastic disease with liver metastases: the Charing Cross experience. Br J Obstet Gynaecol 1997;104(1):105–9.

[96] DuBeshter B, Berkowitz RS, Goldstein DP, et al. Analysis of treatment failure in high-risk metastatic gestational trophoblastic disease. Gynecol Oncol 1988;29(2):199–207.

[97] Evans Jr AC, Soper JT, Clarke-Pearson DL, et al. Gestational trophoblastic disease metastatic to the central nervous system. Gynecol Oncol 1995;59(2):226–30.

[98] Ilancheran A, Ratnam SS, Baratham G. Metastatic cerebral choriocarcinoma with primary neurological presentation. Gynecol Oncol 1988;29(3):361–4.

[99] Jones WB, Cardinale C, Lewis Jr JL. Management of high-risk gestational trophoblastic disease–the Memorial Hospital experience. Int J Gynecol Cancer 1997;7(1):27–33.

[100] Small Jr W, Lurain JR, Shetty RM, et al. Gestational trophoblastic disease metastatic to the brain. Radiology 1996;200(1):277–80.

[101] Kang SB, Lee CM, Kim JW, et al. Chemo-resistant choriocarcinoma cured by pulmonary lobectomy and craniotomy. Int J Gynecol Cancer 2000;10(2):165–9.

[102] Newlands ES, Holden L, Seckl MJ, et al. Management of brain metastases in patients with high-risk gestational trophoblastic tumors. J Reprod Med 2002;47(6):465–71.

[103] Ikeda I, Miura T, Kondo I, et al. Metastatic choriocarcinoma of the kidney discovered by refractory hematuria. Hinyokika Kiyo 1996;42(6):447–9.

[104] Wang YE, Song HZ, Yang XY, et al. Renal metastases of choriocarcinoma. A clinicopathological study of 31 cases. Chin Med J (Engl) 1991;104(9):716–20.

[105] Berkowitz RS, Osathanondh R, Goldstein DP, et al. Cerebrospinal fluid human chorionic gonadotropin levels in normal pregnancy and choriocarcinoma. Surg Gynecol Obstet 1981; 153(5):687–9.

[106] Bakri Y, al-Hawashim N, Berkowitz R. CSF/serum beta-hCG ratio in patients with brain metastases of gestational trophoblastic tumor. J Reprod Med 2000;45(2):94–6.

[107] Bagshawe KD, Harland S. Immunodiagnosis and monitoring of gonadotrophin-producing metastases in the central nervous system. Cancer 1976;38(1):112–8.

[108] Bower M, Newlands ES, Holden L, et al. EMA/CO for high-risk gestational trophoblastic tumors: results from a cohort of 272 patients. J Clin Oncol 1997;15(7):2636–43.

[109] Dgani R, Zalel Y, Biran H, et al. Successful resolution of persistent trophoblastic disease after partial mole with the EMA-CO regimen. Eur J Obstet Gynecol Reprod Biol 1994;54(1):77–9.

[110] Escobar PF, Lurain JR, Singh DK, et al. Treatment of high-risk gestational trophoblastic neoplasia with etoposide, methotrexate, actinomycin D, cyclophosphamide, and vincristine chemotherapy. Gynecol Oncol 2003;91(3):552–7.

[111] Au WY, Ma SK, Chung LP, et al. Two cases of therapy-related acute promyelocytic leukemia (t-APL) after mantle cell lymphoma and gestational trophoblastic disease. Ann Hematol 2002; 81(11):659–61.

[112] van der Houwen C, Rietbroek RC, Lok CA, et al. Feasibility of central co-ordinated EMA/CO for gestational trophoblastic disease in the Netherlands. BJOG 2004;111(2):143–7.

[113] Kushner BH, Heller G, Cheung NK, et al. High risk of leukemia after short-term dose-intensive chemotherapy in young patients with solid tumors. J Clin Oncol 1998;16(9):3016–20.

[114] Houck W, Abonour R, Vance G, et al. Secondary leukemias in refractory germ cell tumor patients undergoing autologous stem-cell transplantation using high-dose etoposide. J Clin Oncol 2004;22(11):2155–8.

[115] Lurain JR, Nejad B. Secondary chemotherapy for high-risk gestational trophoblastic neoplasia. Gynecol Oncol 2005;97(2):618–23.

[116] Markman M. Experience with platinum-based and high-dose chemotherapy in patients with gestational trophoblastic disease: possible implications for future management. J Cancer Res Clin Oncol 2004;130(7):383–7.

[117] Lotz JP, Andre T, Bouleuc C, et al. The ICE regimen (ifosfamide, carboplatin, etoposide) for the treatment of germ-cell tumors and metastatic trophoblastic disease. Bone Marrow Transplant 1996;18(Suppl 1):S55–9.

[118] Piamsomboon S, Kudelka AP, Termrungruanglert W, et al. Remission of refractory gestational trophoblastic disease in the brain with ifosfamide, carboplatin, and etoposide (ICE): first report and review of literature. Eur J Gynaecol Oncol 1997;18(6):453–6.

[119] Sutton GP, Soper JT, Blessing JA, et al. Ifosfamide alone and in combination in the treatment of refractory malignant gestational trophoblastic disease. Am J Obstet Gynecol 1992;167(2): 489–95.

[120] van Besien K, Verschraegen C, Mehra R, et al. Complete remission of refractory gestational trophoblastic disease with brain metastases treated with multicycle ifosfamide, carboplatin, and etoposide (ICE) and stem cell rescue. Gynecol Oncol 1997;65(2):366–9.

[121] Jones WB, Schneider J, Shapiro F, et al. Treatment of resistant gestational choriocarcinoma with taxol: a report of two cases. Gynecol Oncol 1996;61(1):126–30.

[122] Joshua AM, Carter JR, Beale P. The use of taxanes in choriocarcinoma; a case report and review of the literature. Gynecol Oncol 2004;94(2):581–3.

[123] Osborne R, Covens A, Merchandani DE, et al. Successful salvage of relapsed high-risk gestational trophoblastic neoplasia patients using a novel paclitaxel-containing doublet. J Reprod Med 2004;49(8):655–61.

[124] Termrungruanglert W, Kudelka AP, Piamsomboon S, et al. Remission of refractory gestational trophoblastic disease with high-dose paclitaxel. Anticancer Drugs 1996;7(5):503–6.

[125] Farghaly SA. A possible chemotherapeutic response by paclitaxel and other antineoplastic agents in treatment of choriocarcinoma in vitro. Am J Obstet Gynecol 1996;175(4 Pt 1): 1075–7.

[126] Marth C, Lang T, Widschwendter M, et al. Effects of taxol on choriocarcinoma cells. Am J Obstet Gynecol 1995;173(6):1835–42.

[127] Olesnicky G, Quinn M. Molar pregnancy after artificial insemination (donor). Lancet 1984; 1(8389):1296.

[128] Bruchim I, Kidron D, Amiel A, et al. Complete hydatidiform mole and a coexistent viable fetus: report of two cases and review of the literature. Gynecol Oncol 2000;77(1):197–202.

[129] Dalrymple C, Russell P, Murray J. Coexistent complete and partial hydatidiform moles in a twin pregnancy. J Obstet Gynaecol 1995;21(4):325–30.

[130] Benirschke K, Spinosa JC, McGinniss MJ, et al. Partial molar transformation of the placenta of presumably monozygotic twins. Pediatr Dev Pathol 2000;3(1):95–100.

[131] Vaisbuch E, Ben-Arie A, Dgani R, et al. Twin pregnancy consisting of a complete hydatidiform mole and co-existent fetus: report of two cases and review of literature. Gynecol Oncol 2005; 98(1):19–23.

[132] Ohama K, Ueda K, Okamoto E, et al. Two cases of dizygotic twins with androgenetic mole and normal conceptus. Hiroshima J Med Sci 1985;34(4):371–5.

[133] Altaras MM, Rosen DJ, Ben-Nun I, et al. Hydatidiform mole coexisting with a fetus in twin gestation following gonadotrophin induction of ovulation. Hum Reprod 1992;7(3):429–31.

[134] Adachi N, Ihara Y, Ito H, et al. Two cases of twin pregnancy with complete hydatidiform mole and coexistent fetus. Nippon Sanka Fujinka Gakkai Zasshi 1992;44(11):1463–6.

[135] Pal L, Toth TL, Leykin L, et al. High incidence of triploidy in in-vitro fertilized oocytes from a patient with a previous history of recurrent gestational trophoblastic disease. Hum Reprod 1996;11(7):1529–32.

[136] Tanos V, Meirow D, Reubinoff BE, et al. Recurrent gestational trophoblastic disease following in-vitro fertilization. Hum Reprod 1994;9(11):2010–3.

[137] Barriere P, Lopes P, Mollat F, et al. Molar pregnancy after artificial homologous insemination for retrograde ejaculation. Lancet 1984;2(8403):635.

[138] Steller MA, Genest DR, Bernstein MR, et al. Natural history of twin pregnancy with complete hydatidiform mole and coexisting fetus. Obstet Gynecol 1994;83(1):35–42.

[139] Vandeginste S, Vergote IB, Hanssens M, et al. Malignant trophoblastic disease following a twin pregnancy consisting of a complete hydatiform mole and a normal fetus and placenta. A case report. Eur J Gynaecol Oncol 1999;20(2):105–7.

[140] Chamberlain G. Hydatidiform mole in twin pregnancy. Am J Obstet Gynecol 1963;87:140–2.

[141] Gillespie AM, Kumar S, Hancock BW. Treatment of persistent trophoblastic disease later than 6 months after diagnosis of molar pregnancy. Br J Cancer 2000;82(8):1393–5.

[142] Matsui H, Sekiya S, Hando T, et al. Hydatidiform mole coexistent with a twin live fetus: a national collaborative study in Japan. Hum Reprod 2000;15(3):608–11.

[143] Sebire NJ, Foskett M, Paradinas FJ, et al. Outcome of twin pregnancies with complete hydatidiform mole and healthy co-twin. Lancet 2002;359(9324):2165–6.

[144] Coonrod DV, Hickok DE, Zhu K, et al. Risk factors for preeclampsia in twin pregnancies: a population-based cohort study. Obstet Gynecol 1995;85(5 Pt 1):645–50.

[145] Mamelak AN, Withers GJ, Wang X. Choriocarcinoma brain metastasis in a patient with viable intrauterine pregnancy. Case report. J Neurosurg 2002;97(2):477–81.

[146] McNally OM, Tran M, Fortune D, et al. Successful treatment of mother and baby with metastatic choriocarcinoma. Int J Gynecol Cancer 2002;12(4):394–8.

[147] Picone O, Castaigne V, Ede C, et al. Cerebral metastases of a choriocarcinoma during pregnancy. Obstet Gynecol 2003;102(6):1380–3.

[148] Berkowitz RS, Bernstein MR, Laborde O, et al. Subsequent pregnancy experience in patients with gestational trophoblastic disease. New England Trophoblastic Disease Center, 1965–1992. J Reprod Med 1994;39(3):228–32.

[149] Berkowitz RS, Im SS, Bernstein MR, et al. Gestational trophoblastic disease. Subsequent pregnancy outcome, including repeat molar pregnancy. J Reprod Med 1998;43(1):81–6.

[150] Lok CA, van der Houwen C, ten Kate-Booij MJ, et al. Pregnancy after EMA/CO for gestational trophoblastic disease: a report from The Netherlands. BJOG 2003;110(6):560–6.

[151] Zhu L, Song H, Yang X, et al. Pregnancy outcome of patients conceiving within one year after chemotherapy for gestational trophoblastic tumor: a clinical report of 22 cases. Chin Med J (Engl) 1998;111(11):1004–6.

[152] Tuncer ZS, Bernstein MR, Goldstein DP, et al. Outcome of pregnancies occurring before completion of human chorionic gonadotropin follow-up in patients with persistent gestational trophoblastic tumor. Gynecol Oncol 1999;73(3):345–7.

[153] Fallahian M. Familial gestational trophoblastic disease. Placenta 2003;24(7):797–9.

ELSEVIER
SAUNDERS

Obstet Gynecol Clin N Am
32 (2005) 685–702

OBSTETRICS AND
GYNECOLOGY
CLINICS
OF NORTH AMERICA

# Cumulative Index 2005

*Note:* Page numbers of article titles are in **boldface** type.

0889-8545/05/$ – see front matter © 2005 Elsevier Inc. All rights reserved.
doi:10.1016/S0889-8545(05)00076-8                                    *obgyn.theclinics.com*